Yoga: step by step

Erling Petersen

Yoga: step by step

*– A source book of
classical yoga exercises*

A & C Black · London

This edition was first published in 1986 by A & C Black
(Publishers) Limited, 35 Bedford Row, London, WC1R 4JH.

First published in Denmark
by Borgens Forlag A-S, under the
title *Yoga-asanas*.

© 1984 N. U. Yoga Ashrama, Gylling, Denmark

Photographs: Tom Guldbrandsen
Layout and drawings: Elsebeth Morville

This book is the result of teamwork by the members of
N. U. Yoga Ashrama, Gylling, Denmark.
The photos have been taken in the meditation hall of the Ashrama.
Rigmor Fagerberg has instructed the models, and made her
considerable experience available in the preparation of this book.

The models are: Marianne Tornøe (dark blue), Maja Guldbrandsen
(red), Catrine Marcussen (orange), Tine Meyer (light blue) and
Erik Tarp.

Erling Petersen was born in Copenhagen in 1942. He is the
administrator of N. U. Yoga Ashrama, Gylling, Denmark,
and has been involved with its construction since the beginning
in 1967.
He has made several trips to India, where he has received a
practical and theoretical training in yoga from his guru,
Swami Narayanananda.
The system of yoga exercises, which is described in this book,
is followed in the different centres of N. U. Yoga Ashrama, and
is used by the instructors of N. U. Yoga Teachers' Association.

Petersen, Erling
  Yoga – step by step.
  1. Yoga, Hatha
  I. Title   II. Yoga-asanas. *English*
  613.7   RA781.7

  ISBN 0-7136-5651-4

Dedicated to
Swami Narayanananda

"Health is wealth. A healthy body makes a healthy mind. Practise Yoga-Asanas, Prana-yamas and meditation and enjoy good health, peace and Wisdom."

Swami Narayanananda

Contents

Introduction 9

Chapter 1
Warming up and pre- training 25
Exercises for the neck 26
Exercises for the eyes 28
Exercises for the shoulders 30
Exercises for the back 34
Exercises for the abdominal muscles 38
Exercises for the legs and feet 40
Hand exercises 46

Chapter 2
Yoga-asanas 47
Sirshasana 49
Sarvangasana 54
Viparita karani 57
Halasana 58
Matsyasana 60
Bhujangasana 62
Salabhasana 64
Dhanurasana 66
Ardha matsyendrasana 68
Paschimottanasana 70
Mayurasana 72
Supta vajrasana 74
Janu sirshasana 76
Chakrasana 78
Kandharasana 80
Kurmasana 81
Pavanamuktasana 82
Hanumanasana 83
Gomukhasana 84
Chatuskonasana 86
Akarna dhanurasana 87
Samkatasana 88
Mandukasana 90
Kutilangasana 91
Ustrasana 92
Setuasana 94
Uttan pristhasana 95
Simhasana 96
Vajrasana 97
Ardha chandrasana 98
Garudasana 100
Vrikshasana 101
Natarajasana 102

Trikonasana 104
Utkatasana 106
Bhadrasana 107
Savasana 108
Meditation postures 110
Padmasana 112
Yoga Mudra 114
Suryanamaskar 116

Chapter 3
Mudras and bandhas 119
Jalandhara bandha 120
Mula bandha 120
Uddiyana bandha 121
Maha mudra 122
Maha bandha 123
Maha veda 124

Chapter 4
Breathing exercises 125
The complete breath 126
Wave breathing 128
Pranayama No. 1 129

Chapter 5
Concentration exercises 131
Trataka 132
Concentration on sound 133
Concentration on void 133

Chapter 6
Exercise series 135
No. 1 136
No. 2 137
No. 3 138
No. 4 139
No. 5 140
No. 6 141
No. 7 142
No. 8 143
No. 9 144

Supplement
Anatomical atlas 145
Glossary 157
Bibliography 159

Introduction

Yoga-asanas is the common name for a number of physical exercises which form a part of the Indian system of yoga. These exercises are performed in order to attain the best possible state of health together with a deep relaxation of both body and mind. In classical yoga however, physical health is not perceived as an aim in itself, but as a means to higher spiritual development. Yogic physical exercises were therefore originally performed as a preparatory and supplementary training to more advanced breathing and meditative exercises. Today, the practice of yoga is no longer limited to initiated spiritual aspirants, but has become accessible to all. Yoga-asanas have become particularly popular, and they are often done with the limited aim of physical health only. In this book we have not described yoga-asanas as part of either a physical or spiritual discipline, but have simply given them in a neutral, instructive way that can be beneficially used by all.

Yoga-asanas differ from most other physical exercises both in execution and effect. As a rule, a yoga-asana is a static posture of the body in which one consciously regulates the breath and concentrates the mind in tune with the particular character of the asana. In this way, one consciously makes the body, breath and mind take an active role in the exercise, and thereby one gets a deep, all-round beneficial effect on the whole psychosomatic structure. Thus, in yoga-asanas one does not aim to develop any particular kind of muscular strength, condition or flexibility, but a state in which the body and mind remain in balanced harmony under all circumstances.

Regardless of your reason for practice, whether it is part of a spiritual discipline, therapeutic training, or simply for physical exercise, the asanas are the same, and should be performed with equal care and regularity. Carelessly and wrongly done, yoga-asanas will not give you real, deep and penetrating benefit, but may even be harmful. It is therefore important to be careful from the start and take time to learn the exercises correctly, even if it is sometimes a little boring and fussy. The instructions given for each asana in this book are based on experiences with the classical yoga tradition. If you follow the text and illustrations carefully, you will certainly enjoy a wonderful improvement in your physical and mental health.

The Body

Apart from the motionless posture of the body, a yoga-asana also includes different phases and well defined movements. Thus most asanas comprise three separate phases called the entry phase, the static phase and the exit phase.

The entry phase
The entry phase is the first part of an asana. In this phase the body is placed in the starting position and slowly moved into the final posture. The entry phase is of vital importance to make the static phase correct. If the entry phase is not done carefully the posture may be distorted, resulting in tensions, pain and other harmful effects.

The static phase
The static phase is the final motionless posture of the body, which is the actual asana. In this phase the body is kept in the position for a certain length of time, while one tries to use only the necessary muscles and let the body remain as steady and relaxed as possible. This is the most important phase of the asana, in which the posture should be allowed to exercise its effect on the body without any disturbances.

The exit phase
The exit phase is the last part of the asana, in which the body is brought back to a neutral, relaxed position. This part of the yoga-asana often covers the movements of the entry phase in a reverse order. It is important to perform the exit phase properly to ensure that the body is left in a relaxed state so that the organism may fully absorb the effects of the exercise.

The influences of asanas
While doing yoga-asanas, the body is exposed to a number of different kinds of influences, which either directly or indirectly affect the whole system. The effects of the exercises are due partly to a single kind of influence as, for example, stretching, pressure or relaxation, and partly to a combination of these.

Stretching
Stretching the body is a natural and spontaneous kind of exercise which most people and even animals do to remove stiffness. Morning stretching after getting up, or stretching after a prolonged time in any position, are typical examples. This kind of stretching can be comfortably done by all, but does not reach very deep. Most of the yoga-asanas differ from these by stretching the body in a penetrating way which cannot be achieved by other means.

The muscles of the body work alternately by way of contraction and relaxation. Often the muscles do not relax properly after having been in motion, but remain in a state of tension which gradually makes the tissues stiff, painful and shortened. These muscular tensions may come from cold, draught, overstrain, stress, etc. Many people live in a permanent state of tension which is not only exhausting and painful, but in the long run a cause of much suffering and chronic disease.

Yogic stretching exercises work effectively against muscular tension. It is the stretching effect that makes the body light and supple, thus correcting poor posture which makes the body stiff and uncomfortable. Supple back muscles ease the pressure on the spinal column and reduce wear on the cartilage discs in between the vertebrae. Properly stretched muscles work smoothly, relax easily and respond to a minimum of nerve impulses. All these will cause a reduced consumption of energy in muscular activity and increase the strength and endurance of a person. When the body is thoroughly stretched and relaxed, a lot of vitality is being released through the system, you feel alert and light, enjoy a healthy appetite and good digestion and need less sleep.

With many tense people, even the respiratory muscles have become somehow inflexible, like a kind of straitjacket, making breathing an exhausting and energy-consuming activity. Try some of the yoga exercises that stretch the abdominal and respiratory muscles and notice how free and smooth-flowing breathing becomes and feel how the breath itself circulates energy and well-being throughout the whole body.

Tense and contracted muscles cause pressure on the blood-vessels and hamper circulation, reducing oxygen supply to the muscle tissues and blocking the removal of waste materials from the cells. The stretching exercises

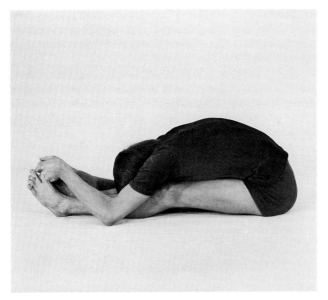

The effect of yoga-asanas

Paschimottanasana is a typical example of a yoga posture where there is a combination of stretching, pressure and contraction. The bending forward implies a stretching of the muscles in the back, while the abdomen receives a light pressure against the thighs. At the same time the stomach is pulled in and up, with a slight contractive effect. The value of most yoga postures is due to this combination of various physical stimulations.

help to drain away all kinds of poisonous waste matter from the muscles and make them relax, thereby easing the pressure on the vessels and improving the flow of blood and the supply of oxygen and nutriments. These effects ease the load on the heart and may reduce high blood pressure. With ample supply and circulation of blood, the cells of the body are kept clean and healthy, preserving the organism and delaying its decay.

Stretching exercises are usually the most difficult part of yoga-asanas because most untrained muscles are stiff and somehow shortened. This hampers mobility and makes it difficult to stretch the body fully in the posture. Stretching exercises should always be done with great caution and require a special technique to prevent painful overstretching of muscles and joints. In the beginning, you should notice how far into the asana you can move the body without difficulty or pain. From this point you should be very careful and avoid violent and jerky movements. Be aware of the muscle groups that are being stretched and take care that they remain relaxed during the whole exercise. When the stretch becomes unpleasant, most muscles automatically begin to contract and stiffen. This point is the stretch-limit which should not be exceeded. To force yourself beyond this point will not increase flexibility, but only damage the tissues and cause long-lasting muscular pain. It is an important rule in yoga that the exercises should never cause pain or unpleasant effects. Pain impulses are warning signals from the body that you should notice carefully. Instead of forcing the body into a painful overstretch, keep it steady and relaxed on the point for a few moments and then, slowly and cautiously, move it a little further into the posture while concentrating on keeping the muscles relaxed. Continue in this way and you will gradually get the necessary flexibility. This process requires a little patience, but it is safe and does not cause any pain. It will also help you to become more aware of the parts of your body which you are exercising.

Muscles and joints should not be stretched suddenly, or stretched when they are cold. Yoga-asanas are easier to perform if you begin with some warm-up exercises. Advanced stretches should not be kept for long, and you should be cautious when the body is moved into extreme positions. Some people are hyperflexible in certain joints and can easily do even very difficult asanas, but they should be careful because a further stretching of the ligaments may make the joints loose and weak.

The pressure effect

In many yoga-asanas, the body is subject to different kinds of pressure. The pressure may be limited to a single spot, or it may affect a larger area. Certain pressures are superficial, while others reach deeply situated organs. The pressure effect is mainly directed towards the circulatory system, the nervous system and certain glands.

Pressure on any part of the body drains the blood away and restricts the supply of blood to that area. This may cause some accumulation of blood in the adjoining vessels and an increased flow of blood through the nearby organs. When the pressure is lifted, there will be a suction effect that further stimulates the circulation of blood. This pump-and-suction effect counteracts congestion of blood, swellings and pain, and promotes a general improvement in health.

Many nerve centres are very sensitive to pressure. A slight pressure, for example, on a nerve centre on the side of the neck (carotid sinus) releases an impulse that reduces the heart rate. Apart from the known physical nerves, yogic anatomy also includes a network of subtle nerve channels (nadis) which flow through the whole body as a vital field of energy. With our present knowledge, it is not possible to give an exact description of what actually happens when the different physical and subtle nerves and nervous centres are exposed to the pressure of the asanas, but it is most probably one of the causes of the increased physical and mental energy that follow practice.

The pressure effect of the asanas on the endocrine glands is likewise a subject of which little is known. Clinical experiments and tests with the effects of sarvangasana (p. 54) and mayurasana (p. 72), suggest that these postures have a regulating influence on the thyroid gland and the pancreas, which are subject to pressure in these pos-

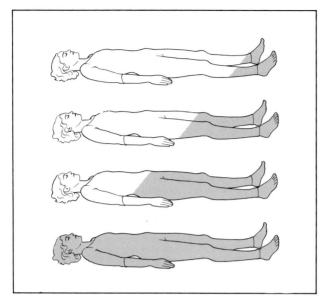

The depth relaxation of yoga comprises both the body and the mind. The relaxation is easiest in a passive, lying posture as savasana. First one relaxes the feet and the large muscle groups in the legs. Then the abdomen, the stomach, the arms and the neck are relaxed. Lastly one removes the tensions in the face and in the fine muscles of the sense-organs. When the body is relaxed, the organism is filled with a peace and a sense of well-being that removes weariness and negative states. A few minutes of real depth relaxation is as refreshing as several hours of good sleep.

Relaxation

tures. It is also the experience of many people with hormonal disorders, that regular practice of those asanas which put pressure on the endocrine glands often helps to normalise the hormonal balance.

Contraction exercises

It is the contraction of the muscles that makes the body move, and as such, contractions are the main element in most kinds of physical exercises. In yoga-asanas, however, contractions are given much less importance than, for example, stretching, pressure and relaxation. In most asanas, contractions are moderate and of a kind that make the muscles strong without enlarging them.

"Mudras" and "bandhas" are the names of a small group of specialised yogic exercises in which local muscular contractions are made to "bind" and "lock" the subtle nervous energy (prana) in that area. But even in these exercises, the contractions are limited and strictly isolated, and in an important exercise such as "uddiyana bandha" (p. 121), a contractive effect is made without actual muscle contractions.

Gravitation effect

Gravitation acts as a permanent load on the body and consumes a part of its energy. The circulatory system is particularly exposed, but also the spine and the breath have to withstand the weight of gravitation. Gravitation means little in most of the yoga-asanas, whereas it is a vital factor in the few inverted postures. In these exercises gravitation works on the body in the opposite direction, with a number of beneficial effects on the system, particularly the circulatory and nervous systems. As the effects of gravitation on asanas other than the inverted postures are minimal, they are described along with sirshasana (p. 49).

Gravitation is a force which we do not normally notice, but during relaxation in a supine position, one can clearly feel the weight of gravity as a sort of pleasant heaviness of the body. This sensation is so closely connected with the relaxed state that it forms an important auto-suggestion in the process of yogic relaxation.

Relaxation

Though stretching exercises have a relaxing effect, they cannot by themselves bring about a general deep relaxation of the body and mind. To obtain this state, it is necessary to place the body in a steady, passive and inactive position which alone makes it possible to become completely relaxed. Savasana (p. 108) is the best posture for the practice of deep yogic relaxation. The physical posture of savasana is quite easy to do, but the process of relaxation is not equally easy for all, and may require some practice. However, if you take the time to learn it, you will be rewarded with a pleasant experience of peace, which refreshes the whole system, recharging it with life and energy. Regular practice of relaxation will ease the unnoticed and subconscious tensions of the body and mind. If you can learn to relax during the stress and struggle of daily life, you can avoid an enormous loss of energy and be able to work harder without getting exhausted. People who systematically practise deep relaxation develop an inner calmness and balance which reduces the harmful effects of disappointments, losses and set-backs. Deep yogic relaxation has a rejuvenating effect, for when we are not disturbed by tensions, emotions and sense impulses, the healing powers of the body can work incredible improvements on our health.

Deep relaxation and yoga-asanas are an ideal combination of exercises that mutually complement each other's beneficial effects. One may say that the postures do the rough work by eliminating the worst tensions and bring about balance in the system. In the phase of relaxation, the effects of the asana get fully absorbed and utilised by the body, while the subtle, unnoticed and deep-rooted strains fade away into a peaceful silence.

Relaxation after yoga-asanas

It is partly for this reason that it has become a fixed rule in yoga always to relax the body in savasana for a few moments after completing a posture. If you fail to do this, you may experience some minor tensions, arising during a number of asanas, that reduce their value. Because of individual needs, however, there is no fixed rule for the period of relaxation in between the exer-

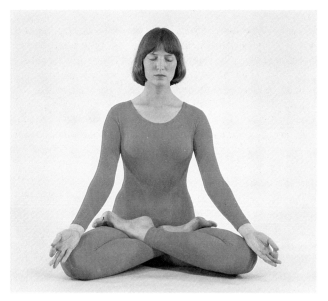

Relaxation and concentration

Although depth relaxation is not the same as meditation, it implies a mental process that may give one an idea of what meditation is about. Depth relaxation is therefore an exercise which often stirs an interest in the meditational technique of yoga. If one practises yoga-asanas and depth relaxation in a regular and systematic manner, it becomes easier to control the thoughts and the emotions, and easier to concentrate. Yoga-asanas, depth relaxation, breathing exercises and meditation are different disciplines that are in mutual harmony, and which together make it possible to develop the best qualities of man.

cises. A beginner usually requires more relaxation time than an advanced student, and strenuous exercises also make you spend more time in relaxation. As a rule, the previous exercise should be "out of the body", so that the whole system, including breath, is brought to a quiet state of balance before proceeding to the next asana. After some practice, this process can be completed in a few moments.

You should always finish the programme with 10 to 15 minutes of deep relaxation in savasana. If you are busy you should not shorten the time of this asana, but instead drop one or two of the other postures, or spend a little less time on each of them.

It is important to protect yourself against any kind of disturbance while practising deep relaxation. Sudden and unexpected sounds may cause a painful disorder in the nervous system, and upset the breath and heart rate. Bright light also disturbs relaxation, whereas subdued and soft light encourages it. Make sure that the room is at a comfortable temperature. During deep relaxation all the organic functions as well as the body temperature decrease, making the system more sensitive to cold and draughts. It is wise to have a blanket on hand to prevent the body from cooling down during relaxation.

Breathing during relaxation

After having placed the body in the posture af savasana, you should begin the relaxation exercise with some deep, complete breaths (p. 126), to make the body still and relaxed. While doing this kind of breathing, try to imagine that each inhalation fills the whole body with health, strength and purity and let your attention focus upon these qualities within, forgetting the outer world. During exhalation you can imagine that you are expelling all pain, illness and harmful ideas, along with the outgoing breath. Such auto-suggestions are very helpful, and in the beginning they are actually necessary in learning the art of deep relaxation. In the description of savasana (p. 108) you will find an easy and effective method of relaxation in the form of systematic auto-suggestions. Try them and take your time to learn the process. Do not be disappointed if success is not immediate. Regular and systematic practice is the key to success in all kinds of yoga. If you continue that way, it is only a question of time before you learn real and deep relaxation.

Thoughts during relaxation

When you begin the practice of a conscious relaxation technique, you may find it difficult to direct the thoughts and imagination according to your intention. Thoughts have a tendency to take their own course, away from the deliberate mental process of yogic relaxation. If you get these problems while trying to learn it systematically, it may help your concentration to get another person to instruct you during the exercise, or by joining a yoga class. You can also record your own instructions on a tape, to be played when you practise. However, when the initial part of the relaxation is over, this connection to the outer world should also be left behind, to allow a complete and undisturbed absorption in inner peace and silence.

Mental experiences during relaxation

In the state of deep relaxation you may sometimes get unusual inner experiences. The sensation of a pleasant, warm heaviness in the body is a common experience that you will get almost every time you practise. Some get the experience that the body-awareness fades away, or feel the body to be extremely light as if it were floating in empty space. Some also see different kinds of light, or hear pleasant distant sounds. These experiences are not harmful or wrong, they only indicate that the mind has withdrawn from the senses and the outer world, and is engaged with its own inner activities.

The Breath

Breathing is usually an automatic process, controlled by the nervous system in accordance with the amount of carbon dioxide in the blood and the need of oxygen in the body. Though the balance of oxygen is thus automatically regulated, it does not mean that breathing also is automatically in good order. Most people actually breathe in a forced and inefficient way, consuming an unnecessary amount of energy and causing poor ventilation of the lungs. A permanently restrained breath becomes a load on the body and may cause increased tension, chronic fatigue, and a depressed state of mind. In yoga, breathing is subject to particular attention and conscious training, as certain kinds of breaths can cause a real and marked improvement in general health. In classical yoga, breathing exercises form a separate discipline called pranayama, but regulation of breath also plays an important role in yoga-asanas.

Breathing is not considered by yoga as only a mechanical exchange of gases, but more as a function of the subtle prana forces, which are the hidden cause of all bodily and mental activities. By learning and practising deep, rhythmical breathing, you can not only improve the function of the lungs and metabolism, but also relax the body, recharging it with energy and allowing a smooth flow in thought functions and the emotions.

The breath reflects different states of mind and emotions. Fear and anger usually make breathing short and superficial, whereas harmonious emotions, such as love and sympathy, cause more placid nerve currents which make breathing deeper and more regular. When the body and mind are at rest and in balance, breathing becomes steady and even. During relaxation the respiratory movements become very fine, and when the mind gets deeply concentrated, breath can hardly be perceived. During the highest state of meditation, the thoughts and nerve currents are focused and absorbed in a single mental point, and in this exceptional state there is no trace of respiration.

In yoga, the relation between breath and mind is being used deliberately to influence thoughts and emotions by means of respiration. If, for instance, you are in a nervous, stressed and tense condition, you can overcome the trouble and soothe the nerve currents by doing some rounds of deep, complete yogic breath. By the simple breathing exercises described in this book, you may gradually improve the automatic respiration also, which will be a real gain for both your physical and mental health.

A breath consists of three phases, which in yoga are called rechaka (exhalation), puraka (inhalation) and kumbhaka (retention of breath). A yogic breath always begins with exhaling, as one cannot fill up the lungs with fresh air without first emptying them. Kumbhaka is a pause between inhalation and exhalation, or between exhalation and inhalation. In automatic respiration, kumbhaka is an unnoticed and very short period, whereas it is the most important part of breathing in the higher yogic pranayama. In yoga-asanas kumbhaka is less important and appears mostly in exercises in which normal breathing is difficult.

Nomal breathing is mainly done by the movements of the diaphragm and the costal muscles. Inhalation is an active muscular process in which the diaphragm is lowered and the ribs lifted so that the cavity of the chest expands and air flows into the lungs. Exhalation is a passive action in which the respiratory muscles relax, letting the chest sink down and the diaphragm move upwards to its resting position.

The four kinds of breathing

Respiration is often divided into three different kinds, called diaphragmatic breathing, costal breathing and clavicular breathing. Apart from these, the yogic system of respiration is based on a fourth kind called the complete breath.

The diaphragmatic breath

In the diaphragmatic breath, respiration is mainly carried out in the lower part of the lungs by a downward movement of the diaphragm. This is the best of the three kinds of breathing, as it supplies a maximum amount of air to the lungs with a minimum of effort.

Usually you breathe in this way while resting and relaxing, whereas tensions in the abdominal muscles restrain this breath. Diaphragmatic breathing has a massaging effect on the organs in the abdominal cavity that stimulates digestion and blood-circulation. The rhythmical movements of the diaphragm have a soothing and regulating effect on the nervous centres of the solar plexus, which are easily disturbed by stress and emotions.

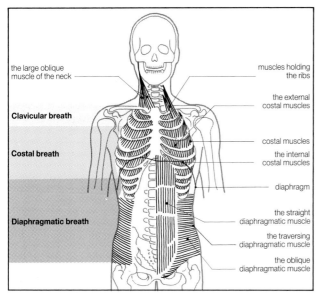

the large oblique muscle of the neck

Clavicular breath

Costal breath

Diaphragmatic breath

muscles holding the ribs

the external costal muscles

costal muscles

the internal costal muscles

diaphragm

the straight diaphragmatic muscle

the traversing diaphragmatic muscle

the oblique diaphragmatic muscle

The complete yoga breathing

Breathing may be divided into three phases according to the muscle groups that one uses during respiration. In the abdominal breathing the diaphragm is active in a way that stimulates all the organs in the abdominal cavity. In the costal breathing the costal muscles makes the chest expand and contract, and in the clavicular breathing the muscles of the neck and shoulders are used to ventilate the apex of the lungs. In the complete yogic breathing the movements of all these muscles are combined in a deep respiration that is felt from the lower abdomen up to the throat. If these muscle movements are combined in the right way (see p. 126), a smooth breathing is achieved which may be alleviating tensions and blockings everywhere in the organism. The illustration shows the situation of the most important muscle groups on the front side of the body, taking part in the various phases of respiration.

The costal breath

In this kind of breathing inhalation is caused by the costal muscles which elevate and expand the chest. Costal breathing is more strenuous and does not ventilate the lungs as well as the diaphragmatic breath. You usually breathe in this way when under stress and tension, or if you are fat or are wearing tight clothing.

The clavicular breath

You rarely use the clavicular breath in ordinary breathing. This breath further ventilates the apex of the lungs by the muscles of the neck and shoulders. This only allows a poor intake of air with maximum effort. As a separate breath it is active only in extreme situations and can be seen as a short, gasping respiration, for example, in weeping or during certain asthmatic fits.

The complete breath

The basis of yogic breathing exercises is called the complete breath and consists of a systematic combination of the three partial kinds. In the complete breath you utilise the full volume of the lungs in a slow, even and rhythmic respiration, thus making the different groups of muscles work coherently and smoothly. Knowledge of the complete yogic breath makes you aware of the hidden subtleties of respiration, and should be one of the first subjects of your yoga practices.

When you begin to practise complete breathing, you may come across a lot of tensions in the respiratory muscles of which you have never previously been aware. It usually takes time to root these out so as to establish a complete, well co-ordinated and relaxed working of the breath, and at first the process may seem a little unnatural and complicated. In the description of the complete yogic breath (p. 126), some methods have been given which are helpful in initial practice. When once you master this breath, it should be practised as much as possible and as often as possible. It can be done by all, in all places and at all times. It will prove quite refreshing and strengthening to do some rounds now and then during the day, whether you are lying, standing, sitting or walking.

It is most important to do deep yogic breathing as slowly as possible. If you do rapid deep breathing, you may upset the balance between oxygen and carbon dioxide in the blood, which will cause giddiness and other unpleasant effects. The deep yogic breathing exercises are not primarily designed to increase the capacity of the lungs, but more to ventilate all the tissues of the lungs and harmonise the rhythmic nerve impulses that activate respiration.

Exhalation

Certain schools of yoga regard exhalation as the most important phase in respiration, because a deep exhalation almost automatically causes a deep inhalation. On the other hand, a deep inhalation will not in the same way bring about a deep exhalation. The length of the exhaled air-currents differs according to the physical and mental state of health. The force of exhalation can be measured by holding a fine thread in the exhaled current outside the nostrils. If the physical and mental health is poor, the exhalation will be somewhat jerky, with a stronger current of air even in rest, whereas a healthy person will have a soft and smooth exhalation with a shorter current of air.

The flow in the nostrils

In the yogic exercises one always breathes through the nose except in a few special breathing exercises. When the inhaled air passes through the nose, it gets purified, warmed and moistened to suit the conditions of the lungs. People who habitually breathe through the mouth often cough and suffer disorders of the respiratory organs.

In ordinary breathing one of the nostrils is always more active than the other one. This condition changes from one side to the other approximately every two and a half hours, and is connected with some very subtle or "wireless" nerve paths (yoga nadis) that interact with respiration and influence our physical and mental energies. When the right nostril is active, the so-called Pingala nadi (Surya or Sun nerve), will dominate with its heating quality and make one more active and extrovert. When the left nostril is active, Ida nadi (Chandra or Moon nerve), will be

Pranayama

The Indian yogi, Swami Narayanananda, is here doing pranayama in his ashrama in the Himalayas. Note the posture of the hand that closes the nostrils in antara kumbhaka (retention of breath with filled lungs), while the arm is as vertical and relaxed as possible without pressing the chest. The shoulders are lowered and slightly drawn back, with a freely expanded chest, showing a maximum inhalation without tensioning in the neck. Note the posture of the trunk with a straight back and the abdomen and the pelvic region drawn slightly in and upward, so the weight do not make any exhausting tensions, and allowing the breath and the nerve currents to flow freely and unrestricted. The legs are comfortably placed in padmasana, that makes the posture firm and steady. This is a perfect asana, and in such postures the great yogis can do pranayama and meditation uninterrupted for many hours every day without the least fatigue. The photo shows the Indian yogi at the age of 56 years.

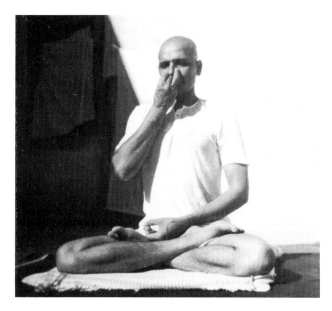

at work, making you cooler, passive and introvert. It takes long practice to notice these very subtle energies that work unconsciously in an alternate rhythm on the whole system. Yogis can change the flow in the nostrils at will, whereas others may do it with plugs or, for example, by pressing a hand against the armpit on the side opposite to the nostril which they want to activate. The harmonic oscillation of the flow in the nostrils and the related subtle nerves are considered vital for the organic rhythm of the body, and the alternate inhalation and exhalation through the nostrils is a basic practice in yogic breathing exercises.

Posture in yogic breathing

The breathing exercises described in this book comprise some simple and easy kinds of deep, rhythmic breathing. They can be done in various lying and sitting positions, provided that the body relaxes and the back is kept straight. If you practise in a posture with a bent back, the respiratory muscles cannot move freely and breathing becomes both strenuous and insufficient. If the posture causes tensions, the body remains in an unsteady and restless state that is both tiring and unpleasant. This also counteracts the slow and even rhythm of the breath, which is the very aim of the exercises.

The actual pranayama is an advanced kind of breathing exercise which should always be done in a sitting posture, usually in a meditative asana. If you practise pranayama in a lying position, you may get drowsy or fall asleep. A lying position will also cause pressure on the back, restricting breathing and disturbing the easy flow of the respiratory process, which requires a relaxed and flexible back.

Pranayama

We have not included any of the advanced breathing or pranayama exercises in this book, partly because it is a separate subject and partly because it may prove risky to experiment with these exercises on your own. Pranayama should be learned individually from an experienced teacher. These exercises have a tremendous effect on the body and mind. They purify the whole system and prevent decay. Pranayama strengthens the nerves and charges the body with a force that cannot be handled

safely without proper preparation. Done correctly, these exercises lead to conscious control of the nervous system, and aim directly at the meditative state of mind. The higher kinds of pranayama are not done for ordinary health reasons, but more as mental exercises that imply a degree of healthy, physical and mental development and a deep, well regulated way of breathing. In his book *"The Secrets of Prana, Pranayama and Yoga Asanas"*, the Indian yogi Swami Narayanananda has given an elaborate description of these advanced exercises and the conditions under which they should be practised.

A yogi who practises pranayama must strictly observe the yogic rules of diet and ethics. A yogi trains for many hours daily in a very regular and systematic way. In this book of Swami Narayanananda you will find a rare description of the highest kind of pranayama, in which inhalation is done in 36 seconds, the breath is retained for 144 seconds and exhalation done in 72 seconds. This kind of breathing continues uninterrupted for a long time in a completely natural state and with the mind so deeply concentrated on the vital power (prana), that even a single stray thought will cause waves of disturbances, making the exercise impossible to do. In these kinds of pranayama, respiration has become so subtle that even a fine thread kept outside the nostrils makes no movement at all. The heart-beats and all other physical and mental activities are at a minimum and the bodily need of oxygen very little. In these exercises man takes over the full control of the automatic and unconscious activities, he obtains control of his sense-organs and brain, and may change any physical and mental state at will. The actual aim of these exercises is to awaken the hidden power of consciousness (Kundalini Shakti), and raise it to higher centres of energy (i.e. chakras) along the spine. When this infinite power awakens, the character and abilities of a person change completely. Such an illuminated yogi is far beyond the normal way of life, with its momentary pleasures and sorrows. He becomes his own master and gets firmly established in the Bliss of pure Consciousness. Readers who want a practical and first-hand description of this subject may refer to the book of Swami Narayanananda.

The mind

In yoga, the condition of the body is considered to be mainly an outcome of the psychic energies, and the attitude of the mind is therefore an important part of all yogic exercises. In the static phase of the asanas, you try to withdraw the mind from the surroundings and turn the attention inward to become aware of the deeper effects of the exercise. If, at the same time, you imagine good, positive visualisations which harmonise with the posture, you can increase its physical and mental value to a high degree. When the mental conceptions become a part of the exercise, the ability to concentrate the mind at will improves, which is a help in meditation and with all other kind of intellectual and mental activity.

While doing yoga-asanas you can concentrate the mind in different ways according to individual capacity and advancement in yoga.

Concentration on performance of asanas

In the beginning of your training it is necessary to concentrate fully on doing the exercises correctly. Asanas should not be done at random and there should be no uncontrolled movements of the body. Try to be aware of the muscular activities that are necessary for the exercise, and at the same time learn to relax all other groups of muscles. It is also important to learn the art of coordinating the muscular movements and to perform the asana in a single, steady and gliding motion, without any jerks. It is this conscious precision of the movements that is the secret of the relaxed ease with which a trained yogi performs the asanas. When you are experienced, the exercises become a natural movement which the body will do almost by itself, so you may concentrate your attention on the deeper psycho-physical effects of the asanas.

Concentration in the static phase

During the static phase of the yoga-asanas, different beneficial and positive energies get activated, and the more relaxed you are, the better chances do these forces have to work freely on the system. If you allow the mind to ramble around with all kinds of thoughts and worries, your body will automatically react with corresponding changes in the physical balance which will disturb the good effects of the asanas. It is therefore important to keep the mind attentive and well concentrated on the inner processes of all the yogic exercises.

Concentration on breath

When you master the physical posture in a satisfying manner, you should concentrate your attention on the breath. Most asanas begin with an inhalation. This is an active process which naturally prepares the body for action. In the entry phase the breath is normally retained, and when the body reaches the final posture, you exhale as steadily and deeply as possible in a conscious passive movement. Now contemplate the breath while in this posture. Find out which kind of breathing is the best, if it should work in the abdomen, in the chest or in the apex of the lungs. If possible, you should always do the complete yogic breathing in the asanas. Let the mind focus on the inhalations and exhalations, and make breathing as easy and relaxed as possible, but never force it to become deeper than the posture permits. In some asanas breathing becomes short and high, and in others it goes low and slow. In some cases even exhalation takes an active muscular move, while inhalation becomes almost passive. Thus there is no hard and fast rule for the manner of breathing in the static phase of yoga-asanas, except that breathing should be adjusted to the individual posture and be as relaxed as possible.

Concentration on the body as a whole

The next step consists of making the mind observe the whole system in the static phase. This should not reduce the inner concentrated attention, but lead to a neutral awareness that only witnesses what happens in the body while in the posture. In this kind of concentration you should not try to influence the system, but leave it to the asana. In the course of this process you may often experience that the body by itself releases a lot of hidden, minor tensions, and that the system becomes more open and receptive to the energies activated by the asana. With such a neutral, attentive attitude, you may get a clear idea of the dynamic interaction between the

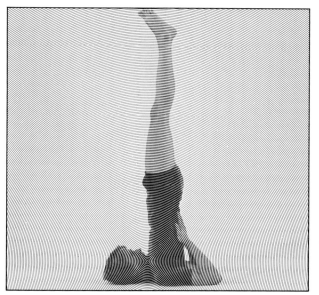

Concentration in yoga asanas

It is important what you are thinking in a yoga posture. Thoughts are subtle forces that influence the organism. Worries are for instance always disturbing in a yoga posture, while well concentrated attention reinforces the effect of the exercise. One may concentrate in different ways according to the individual conditions. Thus certain ailments may be alleviated by the means of suitable exercises and concentration on the diseased part of the body. Sarvangasana (see picture) is a good example of this. Many people have experienced an improvement of a disfunction of the thyroid gland by doing this posture and at the same time concentrating on the throat centre, which receives a particular massaging pressure and an increased blood circulation. Similar cases can be seen in most yoga postures, although there is no hard and fast rule of where to concentrate.

body and the yoga postures, and also a clear awareness of the different parts which are being particularly influenced by the exercise.

Concentration on special parts of the body

Most asanas have a special effect on certain organs or parts of the body. These places vary in different exercises and may be localised by attentive observation of the effects on the body. By mental concentration on these places you can increase the value and make the asanas more effective. The particular place of influence of an asana is not always the same, but may change according to your development. In halasana (p. 58) you may, for example, begin by concentrating on relaxing the back and later find it natural to change the attention to the throat or the breath. Certain schools of yoga advocate fixed places for concentration in each asana, but in our experience, these places differ individually and should be detected by each practitioner.

If you suffer from any kind of pain, tension or disease, you can concentrate the mind on the area concerned, while you remain in the static phase of your asana. This kind of concentration should be done in postures which are beneficial in overcoming your particular problem. When the mind gets concentrated in this way, the vital nerve energy (prana) automatically directs its flow towards the site, and you may feel a kind of warm sensation in the area. These currents give an immediate relief, and if you continue the exercise regularly and systematically it will gradually bring about a permanent improvement of your condition. In a more advanced form of this exercise, you can consciously direct nerve energy from other parts to the place of suffering and thereby further accelerate the healing process. This method requires a good deal of practice and should be combined with auto-suggestions.

Auto-suggestion in yoga-asanas

Auto-suggestion is an important part of all yogic exercises, and in the purely mental disciplines it is an actual necessity in the beginning. Auto-suggestion is not the privilege of yoga, but something by which most of us are often influenced. Strong suggestions can lead to a complete change in our mental and physical condition. It is, for example, well known that terror and imaginary disease can kill a person who is otherwise in good health.

Auto-suggestion in yoga is mainly good, positive and elevating visualization, that harmonises with the exercises it is part of. Such systematic and powerful mental suggestions can intensify the effects of any yogic exercise, and cause a real improvement in physical and mental health. To be effective, auto-suggestion should be done with firm concentration and full conviction. Weak imagination will have little effect and be more like wishful thinking. Systematic, conscious auto-suggestions require some practice. The best way to learn is to practise them, along with breathing exercises and deep relaxation. While doing the complete yogic breath, you can imagine yourself inhaling vitality, health, strength and similar desired qualities, circulating them generally throughout the body or directing them specifically to a localised painful area. During exhalation, imagine that you are throwing out all bad, painful, sick and impure things along with the breath. While thus breathing deeply, imagine that inhalation fills you up from top to bottom, and feel the vitality of the good qualities vibrate in every cell of the body. The exhalation should likewise free you from all painful and negative things, making you feel light and healthy within. To work properly, these auto-suggestions should be practised in a regular and systematic way. You will get very good results if you develop suggestions which can be suitably applied with the exercises and repeat them with the daily routine. In the beginning, these impressions will be imaginative, but after some practice they will become realities that can work wonders on your health.

The effect of auto-suggestion is due to the fact that the mind is a subtle force with consciousness at its back. It has no particular shape of its own, but takes the form of the thought object. For this reason, it is a basic concept in yoga, that what we think, that we become. Our character is a result of the habitual way of thinking in which we live. If we consciously change the character of our thoughts, we can completely change our mental state and outlook as well as our behaviour. It is a distinctive mark of the untrained mind that desires and thoughts

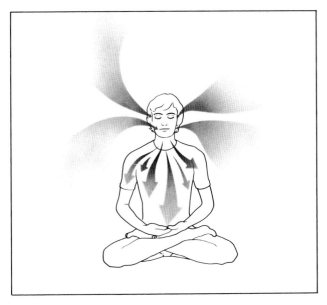

The positive forces of respiration

By means of a deep concentration on breathing, the Indian yogis have experienced respiration as a function of the subtle vital forces (prana). Apart from improving the air conversion and the relaxation of the organism, a deep breathing may recharge the body and the mind with an energy and strength that may cure most ailments and open up to a higher consciousness. In the beginning of the training one uses a technique of suggestion while breathing, which makes breathing comprise the whole organism. While inhaling one imagines, that the body is filled by positive life energy that vitalises, rejuvenates and strengthens each and every cell in the body. While exhaling one tries to feel how all ailments and weaknesses leave the body together with the stream of air in the nostrils. After some training one can really feel these things and experience a real improvement of the state of health.

can easily lead you astray, whereas a well trained and disciplined mind works in a harmonious and elevating manner. All yogic exercises tend towards clearing the mind of negative energies, and auto-suggestion is one of the most efficacious means to this end and makes the mind pure, strong and peaceful.

Thought power

In yoga, thoughts are considered as vital energies which can be compared with electricity or light waves, though they are much more subtle than these and cannot be measured with any physical instrument whatsoever. The force of a thought depends on the strength of its concentration and the intensity of its feeling. Scattered and aimless thoughts are weak and have little effect, whereas a well concentrated and well directed thought is an irresistible power. All people are surrounded by an aura of thought vibrations, which can be felt by others as a certain atmosphere around a person. Even when we are seemingly inactive, we still influence the surroundings by the thought-waves we radiate. All kinds of negative, aggressive and egoistic thought-waves are harmful both to ourselves and others. On the other hand, good, positive and loving thoughts are forces that help both oneself and others. Thought forces can be directed towards any object and will influence it, according to their power and character. With a strong and well concentrated thought, you can harm or help another person regardless of the intervening physical distance. Like radio waves, the ether is full of all kinds of thought-waves, and different countries, cities and houses have a distinct atmosphere which is mainly due to the character of the dominating thought vibrations. When you think a particular thought, you become receptive to the influence of similar thought-waves vibrating in the air. Most people usually emit weak and scattered thoughts, and are easily influenced by the concentrated thought power of stronger persons. By the performance of yogic exercises and meditation, you can improve mental strength and concentration, and make the mind live in good, healthy and elevating thoughts. Thereby you are well protected against bad influences of all kinds of negative forces, and at the same time you become a real help to yourself and your fellow beings.

Mind control

Mind is the actual object of training in yoga. The physical training and breathing exercises are basically a means to bring about peace and harmony to the fickle mind. Mind control is an ancient yogic practice that transforms the whole sphere of body and mind. For thousands of years, the great Indian yogis of each generation have attained a physical and mental state of perfection that rendered it possible to still their mind and senses completely and, in this state of pure awareness they have realised their innermost Self or Atman. This realisation is described by yogis as Ultimate Liberation (Moksha), in which the limitations of individuality are transcended and merge with the infinite Ocean of Consciousness, which is also known as Brahman, God, Self, etc.

Usually the mind lives in a scattered and extrovert state, strongly attached to the sense-organs, and almost every desire, thought and emotion is directed toward sense-impulses. The mind gets its life and power from the very subtle centre of vital energy at the base of the spine (muladhara chakra), which is the dynamo of the physical and mental nervous energies. The sense-organs are described as openings through which this life force (shakti) flows out in a continuous loss of energy. Of all mental and physical activities, it is sexual intercourse that consumes and wastes the greatest amount of vital energy, and in orgasm the very dynamo gets completely drained of its vitality.

Meditation

To regain the original strength and purity of the mind, it is necessary to prevent this constant loss of energy through the sense-organs by turning the mind inward in an attempt to check the countless desires, thoughts and emotions that crowd the conscious, subconscious and unconscious planes. This process is called meditation, and it is the most important discipline in yoga. In meditation the scattered forces of the mind become united in concentration on a single point without thinking of any-

Concentration and meditation

It is outside the scope of this book to describe the real meditation technique, but certain simple concentration exercises may be useful as a supplement to the yoga postures and to make the mind more calm and peaceful. The concentration exercises on page 131ff. may be performed at any time, but one often gets the best result if one does them immediately after relaxation in savasana. Concentration exercises may be done in various sitting postures, but the spine should be straight and the body relaxed and immovable. The best posture for concentration exercises are padmasana and the other meditation postures (see page 110).

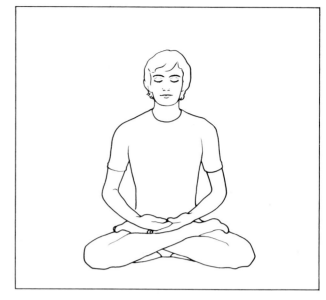

thing else. Meditation can be compared to a strong optic lens that catches the rays of the sun and concentrates them in a focal point of radiant light. The more rays that are united and the finer their point of concentration, the more effulgence and power the focal point will have. If you can collect all the mental activities in concentration on a single point, even for a few seconds, you will get a rare glimpse of deep peace and infinite happiness, that will vibrate in the mind and elevate it for a long time. If you can do meditative concentration continuously for a longer time, and if your practice is regular and systematic, the mind will gradually regain its lost powers and unfold its hidden spiritual and intellectual capacities. When mental concentration is continued without interruption for about 30 minutes, all traces of thoughts and other mental activities disappear, and the mind merges with the pure, unlimited consciousness. This state is called Nirvana or Nirvikalpa Samadhi, and it is the ultimate experience, the culmination of yoga. This state of Being, Knowledge and Bliss Absolute (Satchidananda) which far transcends all human conceptions, is the hidden and unconscious aim of all human activity. As this state is beyond time and space and all mental limitations, it cannot be grasped by the intellect, nor imagined by the mind. A person who has attained Nirvana is a liberated being for whom this world, life and death are lustreless or irrelevant compared with the eternal and unlimited state in which he lives. The few exceptional people who have attained this state are the real yogis, the minds of whom work from the super-conscious plane, and it is such people who have made the system of yoga, and kept it alive continuously for thousands of years.

Meditation is a difficult and trying activity. Mind control is said by the yogis to be as difficult as leading a river upstream, back to its source. But the reward is a permanent satisfaction that is richer and deeper than any amount of enjoyment in this world. It is the practice of meditation and the attainment of mind control that makes a yogi a supremely contented and happy person, who remains in a state of perfect balance, unruffled by pleasure or pain.

The first attempt to learn meditative concentration may be a discouraging experience. Try to close your eyes for a moment and concentrate the mind on a single point, and you will get an idea of the unceasing and crowded mental activity that makes it impossible to collect the mind. When this kind of concentration is attempted, it is as if the mind revolts by intensifying its myriad disconnected thoughts, which makes it a relief to open the eyes again. This little experiment shows the difficulty of meditative mental concentration, and usually it is not possible to make much progress of one's own accord. In most cases it is necessary to get individual guidance from someone fully experienced in meditation. Unfortunately, only a very few people have this experience, and many beginners get poor or wrong guidance.

It is beyond the limits of this book to describe the actual process of meditation. However, certain simple concentration exercises are useful for the practice of yoga-asanas, and to make the mind more steady and peaceful. The concentration exercises, pp. 131-133, may be done at any time, but you will get most benefit if you do them just after relaxing in savasana.

Readers who want a first-hand description of the whole subject of meditation and mind control should refer to the basic textbook, *"The Secrets of Mind-Control"*, by Swami Narayanananda. This book is a source of valuable information and may also serve as a true and practical guide.

Practical conditions

Yoga-asanas are a kind of physical training demanding little forethought. Specially arranged rooms or costly equipment are unnecessary. You need not depend on others nor live up to any particular standard of performance other than your own. Still, there are certain practical matters of which to be carefully aware if you want the full benefit of your practice.

The place

This should be clean, simple and well ventilated, with a comfortable temperature. There should be enough open space to do the exercises without being hampered by furniture or other things. The place of your practice should be solitary and peaceful. Make sure that nobody will disturb you, and that extraneous noises and other distractions are minimised while you are practising. Sudden, unexpected disturbances may upset the smooth flow of nerve currents and cause shivering, violent heartbeats and other symptoms that will disturb your programme. The ideal is to have a separate room reserved for yoga exercises only. Apart from the advantage of being completely undisturbed, such a room will also have a good and peaceful atmosphere which will help to calm the mind, even when you are out of balance and find it difficult to concentrate. Do not let anyone in a disturbed state of mind enter the room, or allow activities other than the practice of yoga there. These things will disturb the atmosphere. Incense should not be burnt during any kind of yogic training.

The time

The best time for the practice of yoga-asanas is in the early morning. At this time the body and mind are rested and the stomach is empty, the air is clean and the surroundings are quiet and calm. Yoga-asanas dispel drowsiness and stiffness from the body, and fill the mind with good impressions and energy and it is hard to imagine a better way to begin the day. However, many are short of time in the morning or may have a bodily stiffness that makes the exercises unpleasant. In such cases the asanas can be done either at noon or in the late afternoon before mealtime. Again there are others who prefer to practise at night because they find that the postures cre-

ate a pleasant, relaxed state making it easy to sleep. Yet to do yoga-asanas at this time is likely to make you more alert, so sleep actually becomes more difficult. Moreover, the stomach is often heavy after the evening meal, which reduces the value of the exercises and may upset the system. As a rule, you should wait at least three hours after a meal before doing asanas.

Thus the time of practice is a question of individual choice which you must decide for yourself, but once you have found a time that suits you, you should try to make that time a part of your daily routine. Such regular and systematic training is vital for the organic rhythm, which gradually makes the body adjust itself to the fixed routine of the exercises. Regularity of practice develops a habit that makes it easier to keep the daily programme, even in periods when it is felt to be boring and monotonous.

The number and combination of asanas

The ancient Indian textbooks mention 84 yoga-asanas, of which 32 are considered important. In this book we have included 40 classical postures of varying degrees of difficulty. This does not mean that you should undertake a daily programme consisting of all these exercises, but rather that you should select a limited number of asanas suited to your individual needs. There are no rules for the number of exercises in a daily programme; usually some 10 to 12 postures will do. You should be able to complete such a programme in about an hour in the beginning, and half an hour when you are proficient.

A programme of yogic training can be made up in many different ways according to the results you want from it. A list of exercises may include postures that promote a general improvement in health, or it can be composed with a more limited or specialised aim. In most cases a daily programme is a combination of exercises that train the body in a balanced and harmonious way. After deciding on such a programme, you should change it only for special reasons.

The more specialised series of asanas are usually done for therapeutic reasons and are often used to promote recovery after illnesses or for specific problems such as back pains, high blood pressure, asthma, etc. If you prac-

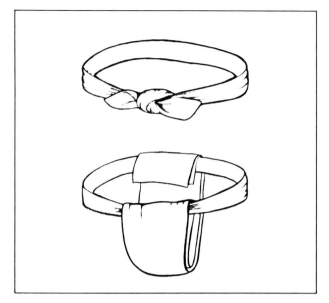

Loin cloth (coupinam)
This simple type of underwear has been used by yogis for several thousands of years. It serves as a good protection of the genitals and the anus, and prevents leakage of prana energy through these organs. People suffering from heat currents, sleeplessness and wet-dreams, may benefit from washing the area with cold water and by using a cold, wet piece of cloth inside the loin cloth pressing against the anus and the perineum. A loin cloth may be used by both men and women as a supplement to the normal underwear, and it consists of two pieces of cotton cloth approximately 20 × 100 cm.

tise yoga-asanas as a part of medical treatment, it should be done only in agreement with your doctor. Therapeutic yoga training is a kind of self-cure which may sometimes replace medical treatment, but it requires some will power and determination to restrict the diet and regulate daily habits. When you are not well it is often difficult to keep up a demanding routine of exercises by yourself. In India many hospitals and medical institutions have done promising experiments with yogic therapy, in which doctors and other experts assist the patients with the practice of yoga-asanas and breathing exercises. In the west, yogic therapy is not so widespread and appears mostly in private yoga schools independent of medical institutions. Yogic therapy is an inexpensive, alternative method of treatment that involves the patient as an active and responsible partner in the cure. This automatically creates a much more caring attitude in favour of a healthy and preventive way of living.

Specialised training programmes are also used in connection with the practice of spiritual yoga. Such programmes need not deviate from those used for general health, except for the prolonged duration of time in each posture combined with certain kinds of mental concentration. Asanas as part of spiritual training may, however, include particular advanced exercises that work directly on the central bodily power (Kundalini Shakti). Such practices should be done only with the help of an experienced guide, thereby avoiding mistakes, which may cause serious physical and mental suffering.

As a rule, a number of asanas should be combined in such a way that a forward bend is followed by a backward bend, a left-side twist by a right-side twist, and so on. This principle will neutralise all tensions that may arise during practice. All rotations and spinal bends should likewise be followed by a straight stretch. In chapter 6 (pp. 135-144), different proposals have been given for the composition of certain general and specialised groups of yoga-asanas which have proved useful for their respective purposes. In much yogic literature of both east and west, programmes and selected asanas for medical cure and recovery are found. We do believe in both the preventive and curative power of yoga-asanas,

but as it is still an unexplored field, we have not taken up that subject.

Clothing

There is no particular rule regarding clothing for yoga-asanas, except that it should be comfortably loose to permit the free performance of the exercises and warm enough to prevent cooling of the body. This point is important, because the system becomes more sensitive to cold and draughts when doing yoga-asanas. Besides, cold muscles and joints become sore and stiff, thereby hampering the movements.

Indian yogis use a kind of underwear or loincloth (coupinam), which is made of two pieces of cotton cloth of about 1 metre long and 20 centimetres wide. One piece serves as a belt, while the second one is tied to it round the crutch. This kind of underwear is hygienic and preserves the vital energy. Many western students of yoga are now wearing this kind of loincloth and find it very helpful and comfortable.

Hygiene

The purification of the outer and inner parts of the body forms an important part of the ancient yogic textbooks. Certain preparatory cleansing and flushing procedures, especially of the nose, mouth and oesophagus are described. These processes are quite efficacious but somehow strange to western people. Apart from these, yoga has little to add to modern hygiene, and we shall describe only two kinds of cleansing techniques that are often neglected in our personal daily hygiene.

Nose flushing

In all kinds of yoga it is important to keep the nostrils clean and open to make respiration light and easy. Usually the nose gets rather superficially cleaned by blowing it, and many people often suffer from blocking of the nose and have to breathe through the mouth. In yoga the nose is cleaned in depth by daily flushing with lukewarm, slightly salted water. This process is known as "Jala Neti," and it is done by pouring water into one nostril, while it runs out through the other by itself. For this

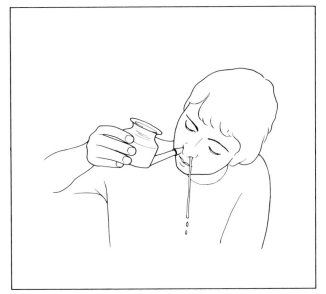

Nose flushing

The classical Indian hatha yoga comprises a series of special cleansing processes of the nose, mouth and intestines. The oesophagus and the stomach may for instance be cleaned by the means of a long piece of gauze which is swallowed slowly and which after some rotating movements of the stomach is pulled out again (dhauti). These cleaning processes are very effective, but require personal instruction. Contrary to these, all can easily perform nose flushing (jala neti), which can either be done with a special jug, or simply by sucking a little lukewarm, slightly salted water up in the nostrils, followed by a moderate blow, so that all water is expelled.

purpose, a special jug with a long, pointed spout is applied to the nostril, the head is lowered to the opposite side and bent slightly forward so that the water flows through and out. This is not a difficult process and can be learned by most people at the first attempt. Do not try to suck in the water or force it out during the process. After flushing one side, repeat with the other, so that both nostrils get thoroughly cleansed. Finally, you can bend the body forward and make a few strong blows through each nostril to get rid of the remaining water. Jala neti done in the morning before yoga-asanas, will give you an improved and easy flow of breath. Regular practice of this neti will also prevent cold in the head and sinusitis.

Tongue scraping

The second process is the cleaning of the tongue, which is usually a neglected part of oral hygiene. The cavity of the mouth is rich with bacteria, which promote a greyish coating of the tongue and a foul smell if in excess. This coating may dull the taste buds and thereby digestion, because the sensory taste impulses trigger the chemical processes of digestion.

The cleaning of the tongue is a simple process of scraping its surface with a metal or plastic scraper. The scraping should be carefully done in a single movement from the root of the tongue to the front, and may be repeated if necessary. Tongue scraping may be done along with cleaning the teeth in the morning. A single scraping a day is enough in most cases, but if the coating reappears, you can repeat it after each meal. This will give you a fresh, clean feeling in the mouth and improve your taste.

Sleep and rest

According to yoga, the nervous centres of the body are recharged during sleep. The more nervous energy you spend during the daytime, the more sleep you need to regenerate. A yogi tries to accumulate and save as much energy as possible, and transform or sublimate it into mental power by means of certain exercises. By learning to economise in the use of this vital energy his need of sleep will be less, and yogis who have developed control over all the nervous energies (prana), need only a couple of hours, or no sleep at all. By the regular practice of

yoga, you gradually become aware of the secrets of the hidden energies and thereby learn to prevent the usual loss of vitality in daily life. Moreover, with a few precautions, you can easily improve the quality of sleep, making for deeper rest and promoting regeneration.

Digestion is an energy-consuming process, and if you take your meal just before going to bed, you may have poor sleep and wake up in a heavy and tired condition. According to yoga, the night meal should be light, and some hours should pass before sleep.

Dreams are an automatic thought function in the sleeping state which also consume energy. If you take heating stimulants such as, for example coffee, tea or alcohol at night before you go to bed, you will be sure to have very active dreams that disturb your sleep. Intense dreaming may actually make sleep an exhausting affair that drains the system of energy. To reduce this activity to a healthy level, the yogis simply avoid anything exciting or heating at night and take a glass of cold water just before sleep. This is a good habit that will help you a great deal to sleep soundly, so that you may wake up more refreshed. Yogis usually begin sleep lying on the left side. This activates the breath in the right nostril and improves digestion during sleep. In the latter part of the sleep they turn to the right side, making the left nostril active. This stimulates evacuation so that it becomes easy to clear the intestines in the morning, a good habit which will also increase your general well-being.

Diet

The dietetic rules of yoga do not prescribe any uniform food for all, but stress is laid on the amount we take, the way we eat and our mental attitude towards food. Apart from this, yoga gives only some general outlines for the selection of food and its preparation.

Moderation is a basic concept in yoga, and to develop healthy eating habits we should avoid extremes and take the middle course. We should take our meals regularly and at fixed times and avoid snacks in between. Do not overload the stomach. The ancient yoga-texts give a proportionate way to determine the amount of food to be taken: fill the stomach half with solids, one-fourth with liquids, and let the rest of the stomach remain

The rules of yoga

The yoga system conceives of man as an individual who is fully responsible for his acts in the sense that one has to go through the after-effects of one's own desires, thoughts and acts. Life is a chain of causes and effects that nobody can escape. In order to avoid painful and harmful effects, the yoga system puts much stress on a sound and ethical way of life which is the very basis of a happy life and a higher personal development. Moderation is a central concept in yoga, and in the holy scripture of India, the „Bhagavad Gita", Sri Krishna says: „Yoga is not possible if one eats too much or too little. Neither is it for those who sleep too much or are too much awake. But yoga can eradicate all sufferings from the person who is moderate in his food, enjoyments, acts and sleep. When one thus purifies oneself of desires and cravings and rests in the Self, one becomes a true yogi".

The ethical rules of life comprise partly a series of acts, one should avoid, e.g. not to harm living beings, not to steal, untruthfulness, etc., partly a number of acts and attitudes that one should practise, e.g. purity of body and mind, contentment and self-discipline. The intention of keeping these rules is not just physical health, but also to avoid all desires, thoughts and acts that entail painful physical and mental effects.

empty. This principle will prevent heaviness and overeating and encourage good health. Avoid too many sour, sweet, bitter and hot items, as well as anything that irritates and disturbs the system. Avoid too much fried food, grilled dishes and rich, heavy and indigestible meals. Avoid refined, over-processed food containing preservatives, artificial colouring and poisonous chemicals, as well as rotten, stale and reheated food. Take only fresh, nutritious and tasty items that suit your constitution. You should adjust your food intake to suit your daily activities, the climate, and so on. Yoga does not promote any particular dietetic system, but leaves it to the individual to solve the problem following the outlines given.

Sit quietly and take your meal in silence. Do not read, speak or do anything else while eating. Be concentrated and aware and take your time to taste your food and masticate it properly. This will allow you to enjoy your meals to the fullest and improve digestion. If you swallow your food in a hurry, or eat when your mind is disturbed, your digestion may be upset and you will not get any real satisfaction from your meals.

It is better to take the main meal at midday, and a light meal in the evening. This will help you to sleep soundly and wake up fresh in the morning.

Fasting is a means whereby accumulated poisons and waste materials from the body are cleaned out. A weekly or monthly fast-day will give rest to the system and greatly benefit your health. If you follow the yogic outlines for a healthy diet, and if you practise yoga-asanas and breathing exercises regularly, your body will automatically be in the best possible state of health, making long fasts unnecessary. If you practise higher kinds of pranayama, it is directly harmful to fast, and in such cases there are different dietary rules to be carefully observed to avoid harm to the system.

Yoga and sport

Though the yogic exercises were originally designed for yogis leading a quiet and rather sedentary way of life, the exercises also make a useful combination with different kinds of sport. In many athletic activities the main muscles often get utterly squeezed, causing painful cramps or after-tensions. In such cases yogic stretches may help in relaxation. Yoga-asanas also make the body light, supple and flexible, increasing the value of any kind of sport. Yogic relaxation may likewise help you to learn how to economise your expenditure of energy and thereby improve your performance.

Chapter 1
Warming up and pre-training

In the beginning many of the classical yoga postures may be difficult to do because of stiffness in the muscles and joints. It can therefore be a help to start by practising some easy pre-training or preliminary exercises that gradually prepare the body to do the actual asanas.

Because of the individual variations in constitution and flexibility, there is no fixed pre-training programme, but when you begin to do the asanas, you will soon notice the areas where you are stiff or weak, and it becomes easy to select the particular exercises that exercise these places.

Many of the preliminary exercises are also good for warming up before your daily yoga-asanas, and a number of them can be kept as a permanent part of your routine.

In this chapter you will find a number of general pre-training exercises, while the next chapter gives the individual preliminary exercises for each of the asanas.

When you do the preliminary and warming-up exercises you should observe the same precaution as with the proper yoga-asanas.

Exercises for the neck

In general

The muscles in this area are often stiff and tense, which may cause local pain, headache, fatigue and reduced mobility, making it difficult to move the head to the extremity. The exercises for the neck make the area supple, improve the circulation of blood, tone up the nerves and remove tension and pain. These exercises are pre-training for the yoga-asanas that require flexibility in the neck.

Neck exercises can be done in bed, before getting up in the morning. Begin with a gentle, circulating massage of both sides of the neck with the fingers. Then do some five to ten forward and backward bends of the head as shown in exercise No. 1 (phases one and two). You can inhale while bending the head backward, and exhale when you bend it forward. After that, continue with some sideways bends and twists of the head (phases three and four). This exercise stimulates the nerve currents and the circulation of blood and makes you fresh and alert. It can be done several times during the day, and it has an immediate soothing effect on muscular pain and headache caused by tension. This exercise gives a pleasant lightness in the head and freshens up mental activity.

Exercise No. 2 is useful for muscular tension in the lower back of the neck and between the shoulder blades. Exercise No. 3 is particularly good if the muscles of the neck are shortened.

The exercises counteract stiffness, but they should be done with care and in a slow rhythm.

Exercise No. 1

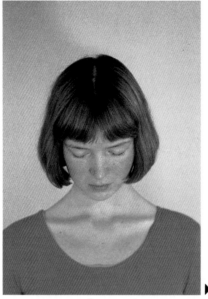

Sit with straight back, stretched neck and lowered shoulders. Inhale, draw the chin lightly in, and slowly bend the head forwards. The bending should begin in the upper vertebrae and be continued joint by joint as far down as it is possible. Then raise the head, exhale and relax. Repeat a few times.

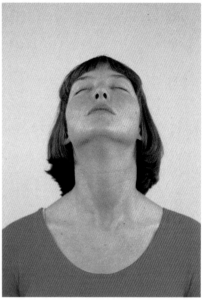

Inhale, stretch the chin forwards, and slowly bend the head backwards. Return to the upright position and exhale. These two exercises may also be performed in one single movement without pauses, and may be repeated 5-10 times with gentle, slow and sliding movements that follow the breathing.

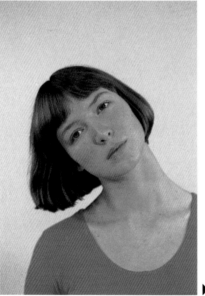

Inhale and lower the head slowly towards the right shoulder until you feel a stretching sensation in the neck. Avoid lifting the shoulder or turning the head. Straighten the neck and exhale and repeat to the opposite side. May likewise be repeated 5-10 times.

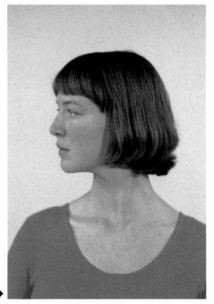

Inhale and slowly turn the head as far to the right as possible, return and exhale. Repeat facing the opposite side, and take care that the chin is slightly drawn in, so that the neck remains stretched during the whole exercise.

Exercise No. 2

1. Lie flat on the stomach, stretch the elbows as far forward as possible and rest the chin on the hands. Relax between the shoulder blades and let the breast-bone sink down to the floor.

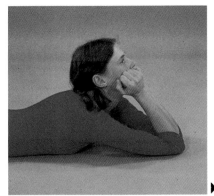
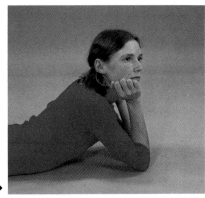

2. Draw the elbows in towards the body, so that the forearms are vertical. Place the chin in the right hand and slowly and carefully turn the head as far as possible to the right. Avoid moving the shoulders.

3. Grasp the back of the head with the left hand and pull gently, so that the chin is turned still more to the right. Look towards the heels. Slowly turn the head to the front again and repeat to the opposite side.

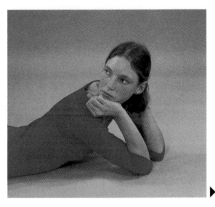
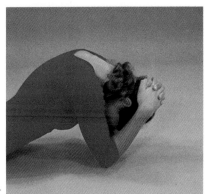

4. Pull the elbows still closer towards the body until the upper arms are nearly vertical. Bend the head and fold the hands around the top of the head. Then press the chin down towards the neck and arch the vertebrae of the neck and upper back upwards. Avoid lifting the hips. Finally relax and place the arms by the side with the cheek on the floor.

Exercise No. 3

1. Lie flat on the back with the hands folded around the back of the head and with the elbows resting relaxed on the floor.

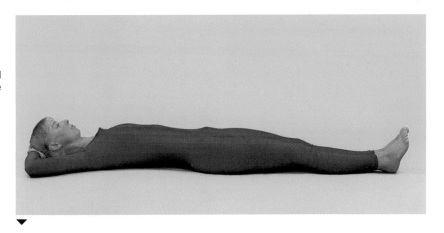

2. Inhale and lift the arms up around the head, pull the chin in and stretch the neck, pulling the head forwards with the hands, so that the neck vertebrae are bent joint by joint. Let the shoulders rest on the floor. Slowly lower the head and arms and exhale. Repeat a couple of times and finally rest the arms alongside the body. Pull the shoulders downward and relax the neck by rolling the head in a relaxed fashion from side to side.

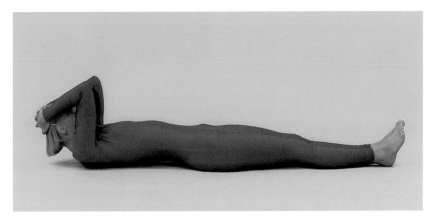

Exercises for the eyes

In general

The eyes are the main sense-organ bringing impressions to the mind, and in the waking and dream states they are constantly active. Most kinds of concentrated work are strenuous for the eyesight, and the eye muscles are often in a tensed condition which may cause fatigue and headache. The eyes are an important means of communication with others, and may suffer strain due to nervousness. Many people find it difficult to relax their eyes, and some easy exercises can be a help in learning this art, thus providing relief for both the sight and the brain. Eye exercises are not difficult to do, but, as with all other physical training, they may cause a little pain in the beginning, especially if you over-exercise.

Exercise No. 1 (trataka) is a "kriya" or process that cleans and strengthens the eyes. First wash or sprinkle the eyes with cold water or weak boric acid lotion. Take a candle light or a flower, or make a dot on a neutral background, or select any other attractive object to gaze at. Do not strain yourself in concentrating your thoughts on the object, nor is it necessary to focus the eyes to bring the object into sharp relief. On the other hand, it is vital to relax the eyes completely and make sure there is no tension in the muscles around the eyes and eyelids. Sit erect and gaze steadily for as long as possible without blinking. In the beginning the eyes usually water after a few minutes, but with practice you will be able to do the exercise for 5 to 10 minutes without any discomfort. You will enjoy the peace and strength that the sight will gain from this exercise.

Exercise No. 2 is a relaxation exercise for the eyes which can be done after No. 1, or whenever you feel any strain in the eyes or head.

Exercise No. 3 is a strength and flexibility exercise for the eyes that combats short- and long-sightedness and gives vitality and health to the eyes. Do not move the head, and keep the muscles of the neck and the face relaxed. Be especially careful not to tighten your brows, when you turn the eyes upward. The eyes should be moved in a slow, even, and rhythmical way that can be co-ordinated with

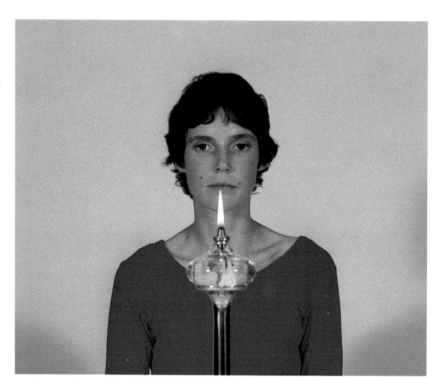

deep breathing. If you have to blink, it is better to do it during the short pause in between the rounds of practice.

Eye exercises should not be done in too bright a light or where the field of vision may be disturbed.

Exercise No. 1

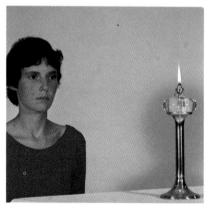

Sit relaxed with an attractive, simple and clear object in front of you, at eye level, and at a distance of about 1 metre. Stare at the object without moving the eyes or blinking. Relax the eyes and the muscles around them. Continue with this until the eyes begin to water.

Avoid straining the eyes in order to focus the eyesight. After some time you will see two objects slightly displaced or overlapping. This is just a sign that the eyes are quite calm and relaxed.

Exercise No. 2

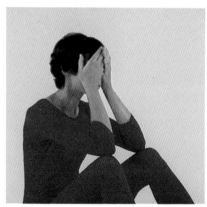

Rub the palms against each other until they become warm. Place the fingers of both hands across each other and cover the open eyes with both palms, keeping the nose clear and supporting the temples by the thumbs. Adjust the hand position so that no light can enter and the eye lashes are clear. Relax completely and allow the eyes gradually to close as the muscles relax. Rest the elbows on the knees or a table. If you feel tension in the eyes, this exercise should be done after all eye exercises.

Exercise No. 3

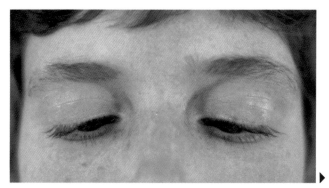

Inhale and look down on the tip of the nose.

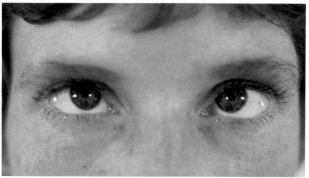

Look up between the eyebrows and exhale. Repeat a couple of times. Look ahead and close the eyes for a moment.

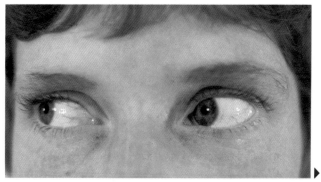

Inhale and look straight to the right side.

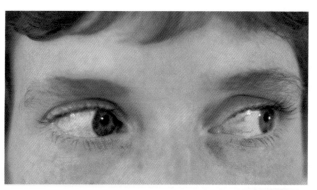

Look to the left side and exhale. Look ahead and close the eyes.

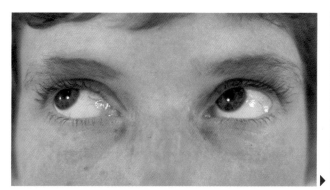

Inhale and look diagonally upwards to the right, then diagonally down to the left and exhale. You may repeat this. Then look ahead and close the eyes.

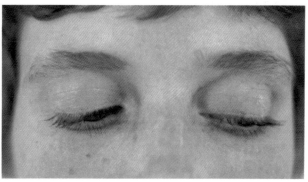

Inhale and look diagonally up to the left, then down to the right and exhale. Repeat, look ahead and close the eyes.

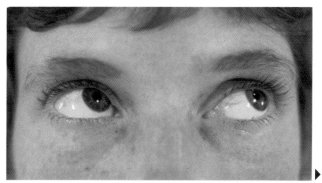

Inhale and look to the left. Move the eyes in a semi-circle along the upper edge of the eye to the opposite eye-corner, and exhale. Inhale and move the eyes back the same way. Exhale, look straight ahead and relax.

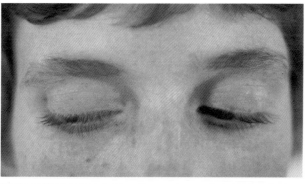

Inhale and look to the left. Move the eyes in a semi-circle along the lower edge of the eyes to the opposite corner and exhale. Inhale and take the eyes back the same way. Exhale and look straight ahead and relax.

Exercises for the shoulders

In general

The shoulder area is an exposed part of the body which is involved in most of the movements of the arms and it is a reflex-zone for psychic tension and stress. Almost everyone has experienced pain and stiffness in the shoulder muscles, and fibrositis often appears in these. Tension in the shoulders may cause pain in the arms, the back and the neck, or lead to a headache and reduced vitality. Tension in the shoulders comes not only from stress but also from awkward working movements and positions, e.g. sitting at a desk, or it may come from draughts, cold, etc. Continued tension may cause stiffness, permanently contracted and raised shoulders which hamper mobility and restrict blood circulation and breathing.

The alternate contraction and relaxation of the working muscles is vital for good muscle tone. As opposed to the arms and legs, the shoulders do not get much exercise unless this is done separately. It is also important to correct the poor posture that increases tension. Always lower the shoulders and expand the chest slightly forward so that respiration is unrestricted. If you sit at a desk or in a car for hours continuously, it will be a relief to do a few shoulder exercises now and then. Exercise No. 1 demonstrates a stretching and strengthening technique for both the shoulders and the arms. Exercise No. 4 is useful if you have muscular trouble in between the shoulder blades. Exercise No. 10 is a true warm-up exercise for the shoulders, neck, and back, which will

benefit your asana and remove fatigue of the body and nerves. For those who do sedentary work, some simple shoulder rotations, as shown in exercise No. 3, will help.

When you begin the shoulder exercises, make sure that the back is straight and the body relaxed. Try to reach the extremity of the positions to make the exercise more efficacious. Be careful if you have weak joints or loose ligaments.

Exercise No. 1

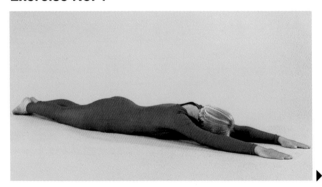

Lie on the stomach with arms stretched forward and forehead on the floor. Stretch the neck a little, so the nose is free.

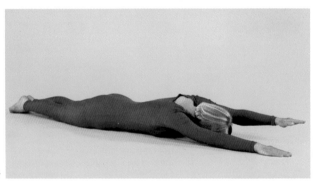

Inhale. Stretch the left arm further forward and lift it. Lower the arm and exhale. Repeat with the right arm. Relax with the hands under the forehead.

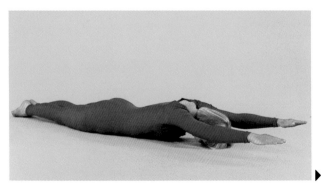

Again stretch the arms forward. Inhale and stretch further, lifting both arms. Lower them and exhale. Relax with arms by the sides and cheek on the floor.

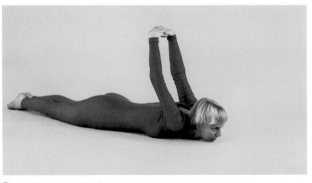

Place the chin on the floor and clasp the fingers behind the back with palms open. Pull backward bringing the shoulder blades together and stretch the arms up towards the ceiling. Remain in this position and breathe calmly.

Exercise No. 2

Stand or sit with a straight back. Stretch out the arms to the sides at shoulder level with the palms downwards. Slowly turn the palms towards the ceiling by rotating the shoulder joints. Twist as much as possible without moving the arms to any side. Turn in the opposite direction and repeat a couple of times.

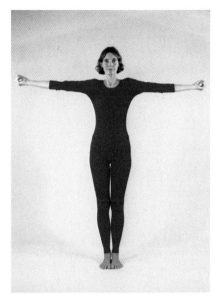 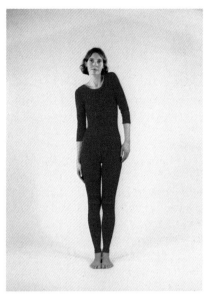

Exercise No. 3

Stand with arms relaxed. Lift the right shoulder towards the ear and rotate the shoulder joint fully. Do this 2 or 3 times in each direction and repeat with the left shoulder. Lastly do some rotating movements with both shoulders simultaneously. Then lower the shoulders and relax.

Exercise No. 4

1. Stand erect with feet together. Raise the arms to a horizontal position and bend the wrists so that the finger-tips point upwards. Inhale and push the arms out to the sides so that the shoulder blades are drawn apart.

2. Exhale and draw the shoulder blades together. Repeat a couple of times. Avoid lifting, lowering or taking the arms backwards during the exercise. May be done with one arm at a time, in the beginning.

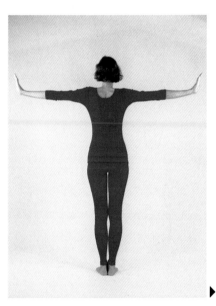 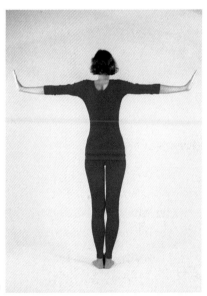

Exercise No. 5

1. Stand with straight back and lowered shoulders. Keep the upper arms close to the body and bend the forearms straight forward, palms facing each other.

2. Inhale and turn the horizontal forearms out to each side and as far back as possible, while the upper arms remain close to the body. Take the arms back and exhale.

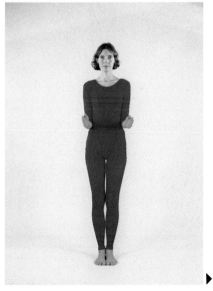 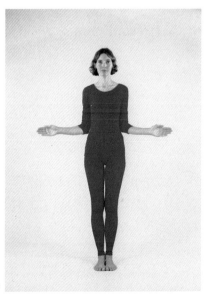

Exercises for the shoulders

Exercise No. 6

1. Kneel and place the hands on the shoulders with the palms facing upwards. Keep the hands horizontal during the exercise and imagine that you are going to lift a heavy weight.

2. Slowly push the hands upwards with resistance until the arms are fully extended. Lower the hands again in a similar fashion and relax.

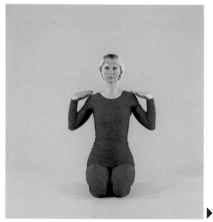 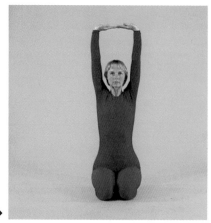

Exercise No. 7

1. Place the finger-tips on the shoulders. Draw the elbows in to the body and take them forwards until they meet.

2. Lift the elbows towards the ceiling, hands behind the head, and rotate backwards so that the shoulder blades meet. Continue moving the elbows down and forward, till they meet again. Repeat twice, then rotate in the opposite direction.

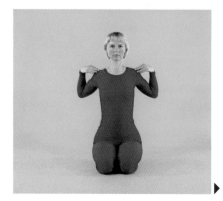 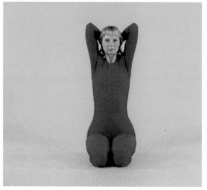

Exercise No. 8

1. Sit in a comfortable position with the back straight. Inhale and lift the shoulders up towards the ears.

2. Draw the shoulders backwards so that the shoulder blades meet. Lower the shoulders, while you exhale and repeat.

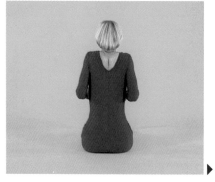 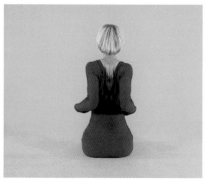

Exercise No. 9

1. Kneel upright with legs together and arms by the sides. Inhale and draw the shoulders up towards the ears. Hold the breath for 5 to 10 seconds.

2. Exhale forcefully while you lower the shoulders and relax.

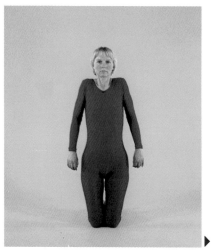 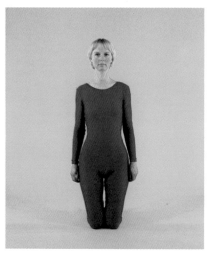

Exercise No. 10

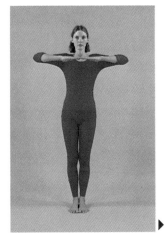
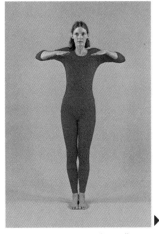
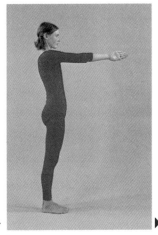
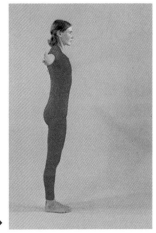

Stand erect with feet together. Join the finger-tips in front of the chest, so that arms and hands are at shoulder level.

Inhale and press the elbows backwards without the hands losing contact with the body. Take the arms forward and exhale.

Breathe in, stretch out the arms in front of you, and turn the backs of the hands towards each other.

Hold the breath and press the arms backwards while they are kept at shoulder level for as long as possible.

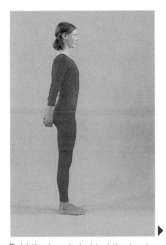
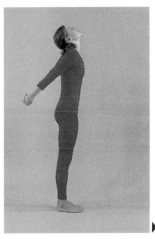
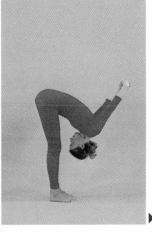
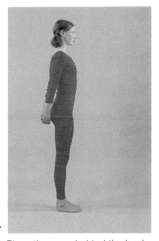

Fold the hands behind the back, lower the shoulders and draw the shoulder blades lightly together. Exhale.

Inhale and take the arms backwards and up. Exhale and bend the neck back a little. Straighten up the head, lower the arms and exhale.

Lower the shoulders concaving the spine and reach down with the forehead towards the knees and exhale. Stretch the arms as far as possible.

Place the arms behind the back, inhale and slowly come up with the chin on the chest. Straighten up the head and exhale.

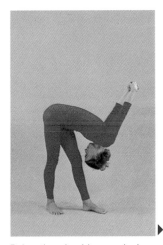
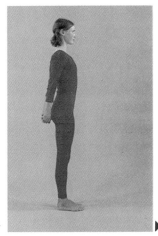
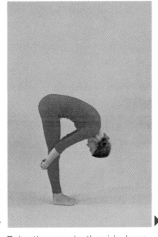
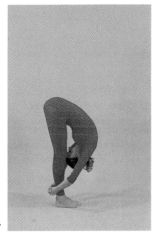

Relax the shoulders and place the left leg diagonally forwards. Inhale and bend forward, letting the forehead touch the left knee and raising the arms towards the ceiling. Exhale and repeat to other side.

Lower the arms and inhale while slowly straightening up the body with the chin on the chest. Lift the head up and exhale.

Relax the arms by the side, keeping the feet together. Stretch the arms over the head and inhale. Bend forward and fold the hands behind the knees. Exhale.

Place the forehead on the knees and let the hands slide down to the ankles. Relax and straighten up slowly while inhaling.

Exercises for the back

In general

In yoga, the back is considered to be one of the most important parts of the body, and a large number of yoga-asanas are designed to make the spine and the back muscles both strong and flexible. By nature, the back is well fitted to meet its many functions, partly as a support and lifting system, and partly as the seat of the central nervous system in the spinal cord. Unfortunately, many people are not aware of the importance of keeping the back strong and supple, and the price for this may include back pain, reduced mobility, loss of vitality and depression.

In yoga, a strong and well exercised back is regarded a precondition for good general health and prolonged youth and vitality. It is important to learn to keep the back straight and relaxed, to avoid soft chairs and beds and anything that may strain the back. It is a good idea to study some anatomy and physiology of the back before starting on the asanas, and in the bibliography on page 159 you will find some helpful books listed.

Back pain has become so common that most people suffer from it at some time or other. It can be benign, and is often curable by changing the contributory causes and by proper physical exercises. If done regularly, the following back exercises will effectively prevent, and in most cases also reduce, the pain in the area. They make the back strong and flex-ible, improve blood circulation and tone up the spinal nerves. These exercises give warmth and comfort to the back, remove fatigue and leave you alert and relaxed. Exercises for the back may be done separately or as a warming-up routine before the regular yoga-asanas. Begin with the easy phases of the series and take up the more difficult parts gradually, as your back becomes stronger and more flexible.

Exercise No. 1 is good for the hip joints and knees. Exercise No. 3 is particularly suitable if you have a weak back. In case of diseases and defects in the spinal column, you should be cautious and consult your doctor before taking up these exercises.

Exercise No. 1

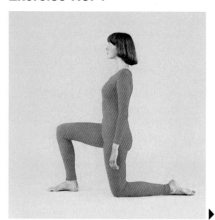

Kneel upright with a straight back and arms by the sides. Put the right foot forward so that the lower leg is vertical with the foot pointing forwards.

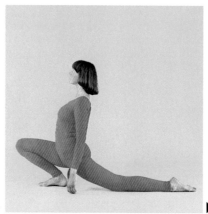

Inhale and move the body forwards, so that the right leg is bent further, while the left leg remains stretched on the floor. Keep the body vertical and the right heel down on the floor. Exhale and straighten up slowly.

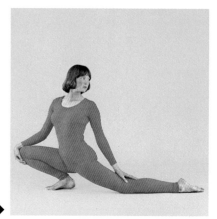

Put the right hand on the right knee and the left palm on the back of the left thigh. Inhale and move the body forwards, keeping a straight back. Exhale, turn the body to the left and look back. Turn to the front, and straighten up.

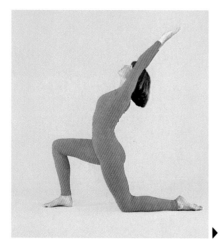

Inhale. Stretch the arms over the head and bend backwards.

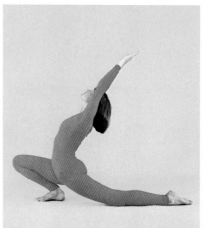

Take the body forwards over the right foot, stretch the arms further back and exhale.

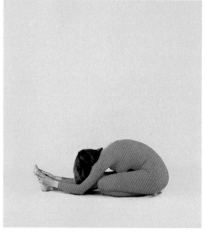

Straighten up and inhale. Sit on the left heel, exhale and bend forwards over the stretched leg. Relax with the face touching the lower leg. Slowly straighten up and inhale. Repeat to the opposite side.

Exercise No. 2

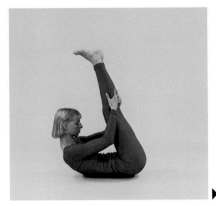

Lie on the back. Inhale and bend the knees towards the chest and stretch the legs up to a vertical position. Grasp the calves of the legs and lift the head. Breathe calmly and make small rocking movements on the middle part of the back.

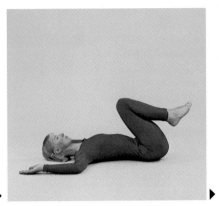

Bend the knees towards the chest and put the arms out at shoulder level with the forearms bent up. Keep the shoulders relaxed.

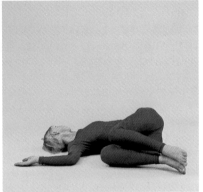

Keeping the bent knees together, inhale and lower the legs to the right side. At the same time turn the head to the left without lifting the shoulders off the floor. Exhale and relax. Lastly return to the centre position and inhale. Repeat on the other side.

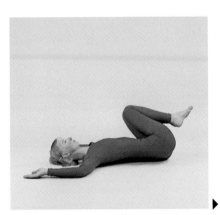

Keeping the knees together, press them on to the chest and move them downwards to one side in a circling movement. Return to the centre position and pull the knees straight up to the chest so that the small of the back is massaged. Repeat twice, and then to the opposite side.

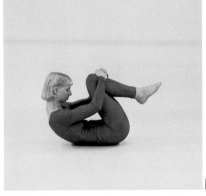

Fold the hands around the knees and inhale. Lift the head and keep the chin on the throat. Make some rocking movements on the greater part of the back. Breathe in a steady rhythm, and take care that the movements do not become unequal.

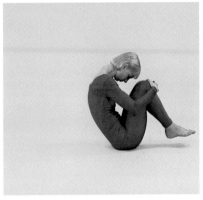

Gradually increase the rocking movements and try in turn to come up on the shoulders and the buttocks, but without putting the feet on the floor.

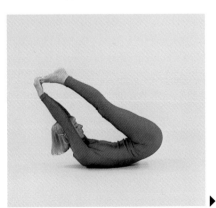

Stretch the legs, raise them and grasp the toes or ankles. Now rock the whole spinal column, following the rhythm of breathing.

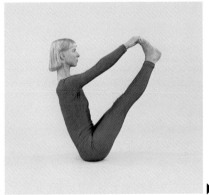

Calmly remain poised on the buttocks. Stretch the legs, the back and the neck and try to keep in balance.

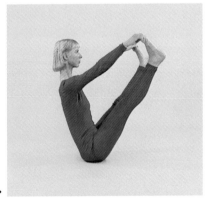

Lastly spread the legs apart without losing balance. Bring them together, relax the back and slowly roll down to the floor.

Exercises for the back

Exercise No. 3

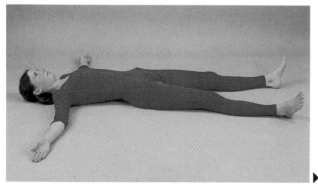

Lie on the back with the arms stretched out at right angles to the body, and the feet separated by about the width of the hips.

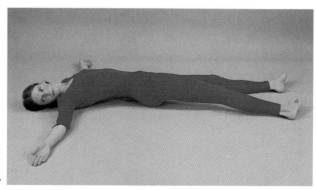

Inhale and slowly turn the feet to the left without lifting the hip, and at the same time turn the head to the right. Exhale, turn back and repeat on the opposite side.

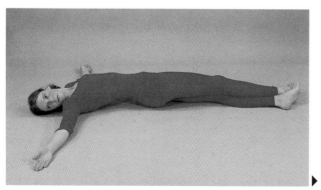

Cross the lower legs so that the right foot is uppermost. Inhale and turn to the left so that the right hip is lifted a little, while the head is turned to the right. Exhale, turn back. Repeat with the left foot uppermost.

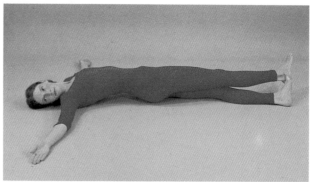

Place the right heel between the first and second toe of the left foot. Do the aforementioned (in third phase) exercise to both sides, change the position of the legs and repeat.

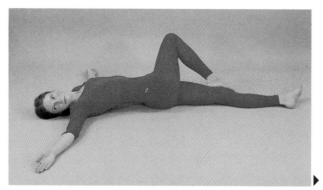

Place the right foot on the left knee and turn as described in third phase. Do not force the raised knee down on to the floor. Repeat with reversed position of the legs.

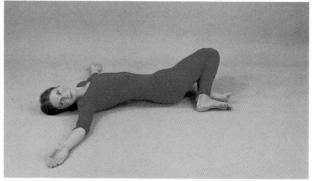

Bend the slightly separated legs and draw the feet up towards the buttocks. The knees are in turn lowered to the right and the left, twice to each side, without letting the feet lose contact with the floor.

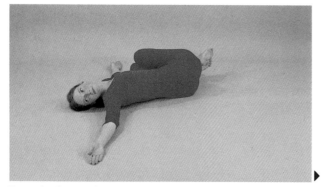

Press the knees close to the chest. Lower them as near to the armpits as possible, in turn to the right and to the left, twice.

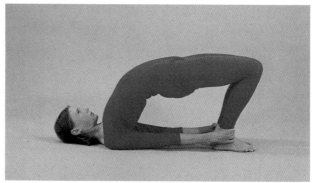

Conclude the series with kandharasana (p. 80). This series is usually called "The crocodile series".

Exercise No. 4

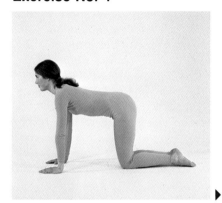

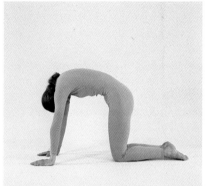

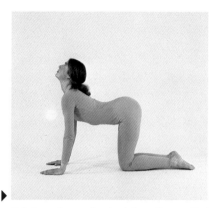

Stand on hands and knees with the back relaxed, and the knees and thighs vertical. Inhale calmly.

Slowly arch the back upwards. Begin with the small of the back and let the movement continue upwards, while the head is bent in between the arms.

Exhale and curve the back from the small of the back upwards, vertebra by vertebra. Bend the neck back slightly and inhale.

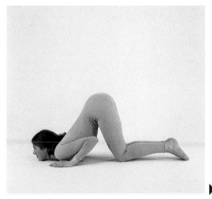

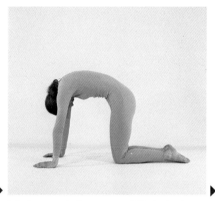

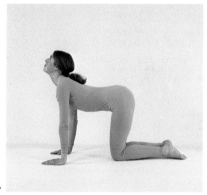

Bend in the elbows and put the chest and chin on the floor without moving the hands. Keep the thighs as vertical as possible. Exhale.

Inhale, stretch the arms and lift the body up. Again arch the back, vertebra by vertebra, and lastly exhale.

Slowly straighten the back from the small of the back upwards. Bend the head back slightly and inhale.

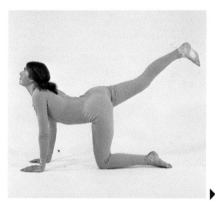

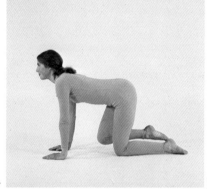

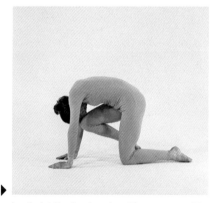

Stretch the right leg back and up with the heel uppermost.

Then bend the right leg and tuck it in under the body. Lift the hip a little and hold the lower leg horizontal and not touching the floor. Exhale.

Lastly let the forehead and knee meet without bending the elbows. Lower the leg and inhale. Repeat the series, performing the last three phases with opposite position of the legs.

Exercises for the abdominal muscles

In general

The front and bottom of the abdominal cavity are bound by the abdominal muscles and the muscles of the pelvic region respectively, and it is important to keep these muscles in good shape. Strong abdominal muscles ease the load on the back, contribute to a proper carriage and may prevent pain in the lumbar muscles. The exercising of the abdominal and pelvic muscles also prevents looseness and sinking of the lower abdominal organs and is a protection against hernia.

Many people suffer from nervous tension in the abdominal muscles. This hampers digestion and the functioning of the internal organs, weakens the diaphragm, and makes breathing more superficial and strenuous. The tensions also increase the pressure within the abdominal cavity and impede the circulation of blood, which may cause congestion. The alternate contractions and relaxations form a vital part of the exercising of the abdominal muscles. The muscles of the pelvic region can be trained by mula bandha (p. 120) and bhadrasana (p. 107). Before raising your stretched legs in the following exercises, it is important to first tighten the pelvic muscles, draw the abdomen slightly in and up, and keep the lumbar region on the floor. Otherwise the internal pelvic pressure may increase too much and you may experience pain in the loins.

This technique can be learned separately by lying on the back with bent legs. Now relax the lumbar region and make a slow contraction of the pelvic muscles and again relax them slowly. Repeat the alternate contraction and relaxation a few times. Do a similar contraction before you raise the legs in the abdominal exercises, and only relax the pelvic muscles when the legs are back on the floor. If you have poor blood circulation or prolapse of the internal organs the pelvic pressure may be eased by doing kandharasana (p. 80) before the abdominal exercises. If you have any abdominal disorders, remember to check with the doctor before taking up these exercises.

Exercise No. 1

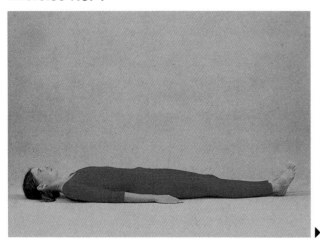 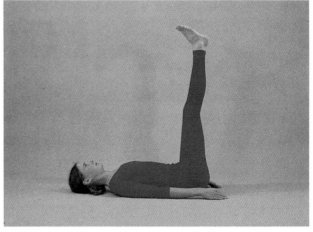

Lie on the back with legs together and arms by the sides, palms downward. Stretch the neck, draw in the chin a little and relax in the small of the back.

Inhale. Tighten the bottom of the pelvis and draw the abdomen in and up. Press down in the small of the back and lift the legs to a vertical position. Exhale. Keep the abdomen drawn upwards and the soles of the feet facing the ceiling. Inhale and slowly lower both legs. Exhale and relax.

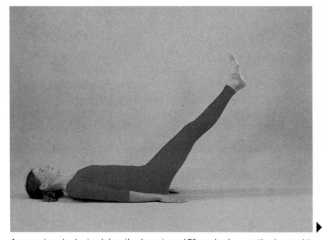 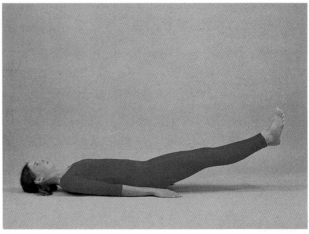

As previously, but raising the legs to a 45° angle. Lower the legs with the toes turned towards the knees. Exhale and relax.

As in the previous exercise but lifting the legs only half as far.

Exercise No. 2

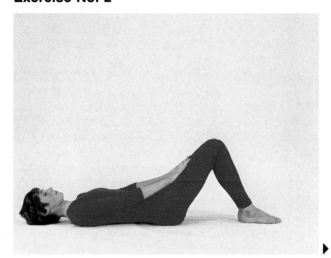

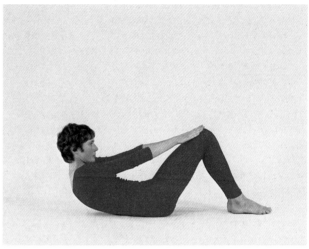

Lie on the back with the legs slightly bent and feet on the floor. Place the hands flat on the thighs. Inhale. Tighten the bottom of the pelvis, draw abdomen in and up and press the small of the back on the floor.

Lift the head and shoulders and move the arms towards the knees. Hold the breath in this posture and slowly unbend down on to the floor. Exhale and relax. May be repeated with the feet closer to the buttocks.

Exercise No. 3

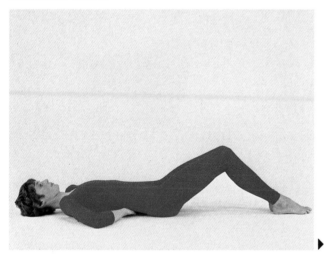

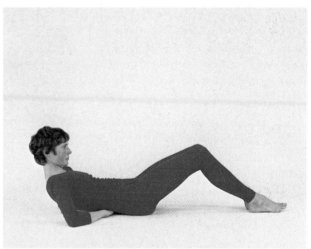

Lie on the back with the legs slightly bent and together, feet on the floor. Place the hands under the small of the back, palms down and with the finger-tips meeting.

Inhale and tighten the bottom of the pelvis, drawing the abdomen in and up. Lift the head and shoulders, support with the hands and exhale.

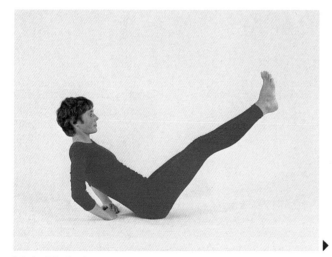

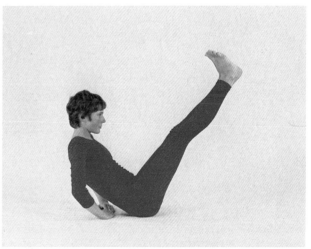

Inhale. Lift the feet until the legs are stretched out, raise the upper part of the body by means of the arms. Let the shoulders remain low.

Lastly go up as far as possible, bend the feet towards you and slowly lower the stretched legs and the upper part of the body simultaneously. Exhale and relax.

Exercises for the legs and feet

In general

Foot and leg exercises increase muscular strength and flexibility and thereby promote the upward flow of venous blood in the legs. By these exercises the vessels retain their elasticity, which will prevent varicose veins and hardening of the arteries. The movements in the exercises affect and train all the muscles and joints of legs and feet, and may reduce swellings, aches, cold feet, and other symptoms of weak circulation.

These exercises increase the mobility of the hips, knees and ankles. They ease tensions, strengthen the muscles and reduce tiredness in the legs. By regular practice they may help to correct poor posture and backache.

Orthopaedic defects, such as flatfeet, may be improved by means of the foot exercises given, which should be done with bare feet. When you are standing erect, the weight of your body should rest on the whole sole of the foot. If you stand on your heels, it will hamper the blood circulation and cause jarring through the spine to the head when you walk.

Exercise No. 1

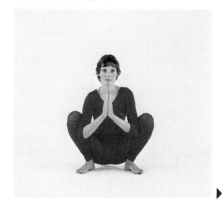

Squat with the feet separated as widely as the hips. Join the palms together and place the elbows on the inner side of the knees.

Inhale. Lower the pressed palms until the forearms are horizontal and the knees are pushed outwards. Keep the back as straight as possible. Relax and exhale.

Exercise No. 2

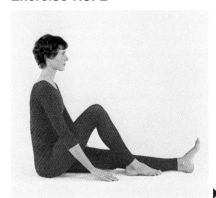 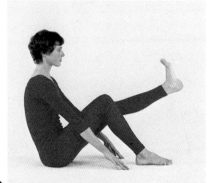

Sit with straight back and right leg bent so that the ankle is close to the left knee. Support with the hands close to the knees.

Inhale and lift the left leg to the level of the right one. Lower the leg and exhale. Repeat with the other leg.

Exercise No. 3

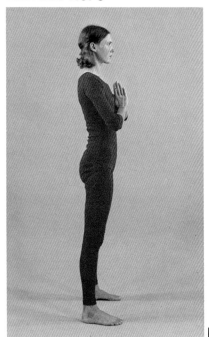 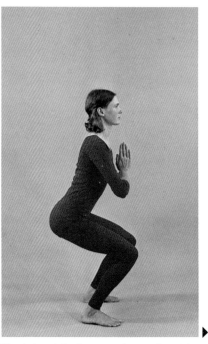 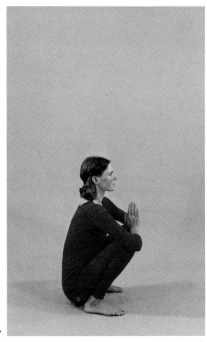

Stand erect with the feet 30 cm apart and pointing directly ahead. Join the palms together in front of the chest and inhale.

Slowly bend the knees and try to keep the back vertical as long as possible.

Go down to the squatting position and exhale. Inhale and slowly straighten up, keeping the back straight.

Exercise No. 4

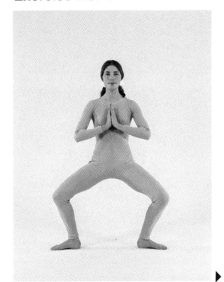

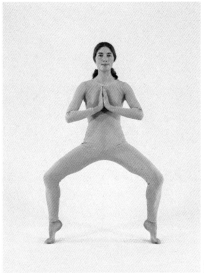

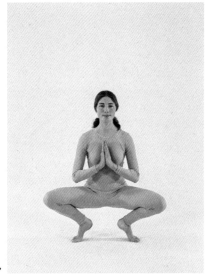

Stand with feet a hip-width apart, toes and knees pointing straight out on either side. Join the palms together at the chest and straighten up the back.

Inhale, lift the heels and stand on the toes, keeping the gaze at a point at eye level. Lower the heels slowly and exhale.

Inhale and lift the heels. Keep the back erect whilst bending to a squatting position without lowering the heels. Exhale. Inhale and come up straight, lower the heels and exhale.

Exercise No. 5

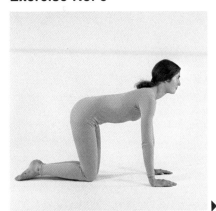

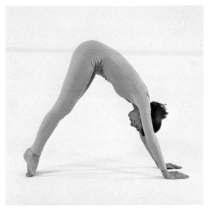

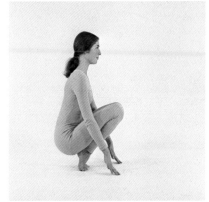

Stand on hands and knees with arms and thighs vertical, toes pointed.

Inhale, lift the buttocks while stretching the knees so that you rest on the palms and the backward-bent toes. Lower the knees, sit on the heels and exhale.

Sit on raised heels with toes pointing forward, keeping the back straight, finger-tips on the floor. Pull the knees close to the chest, and lower again. Repeat a few times.

Exercise No. 6

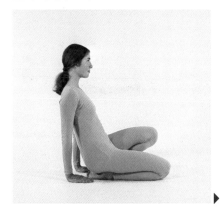

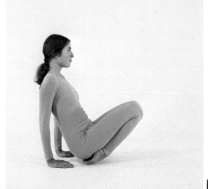

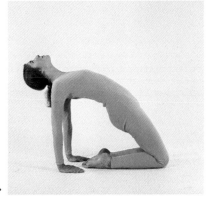

Sit on the heels with knees together. Place the palms on the floor below the shoulders. Inhale and raise the right knee, stretching the ankle. Lower and exhale. Repeat with the left leg.

At this stage one may slide the heels a little apart. Inhale and raise both knees, thereby stretching the ankles. Lower and exhale.

Inhale, tighten the thighs and buttocks, and lift hips and chest-bone high. Bend the neck back slightly. Lift the head, lower buttocks and exhale.

Exercises for the legs and feet

Exercise No. 7

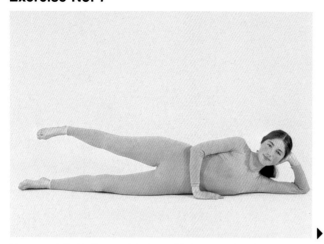

Lie on the left side in a straight line, with legs together. Rest the head in the left palm and place the right hand on the floor in front. Lift the right leg to the level of the hip, relaxing the foot; move it backward, forward and lower.

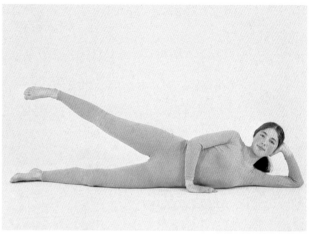

Inhale and raise the right leg to about 45°, keeping it straight. Relax the foot so that the heel is at the highest point. Lower slowly and exhale.

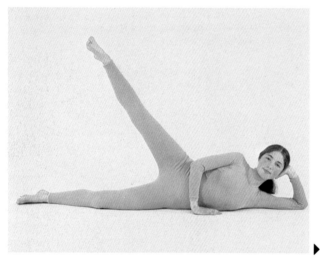

Inhale and lift the right leg as high as possible. Lower slowly and exhale.

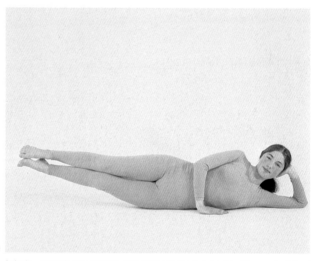

Inhale, stretch the ankles and lift both legs, keeping them stretched and together. Lower and exhale.

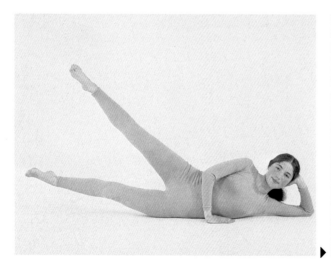

Inhale, lift both legs together, then raise the right leg as high as possible. Lower the right leg to the left one, then lower both legs and exhale.

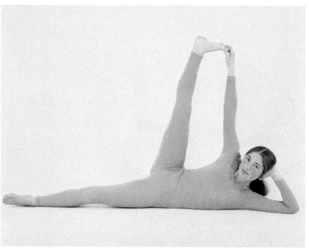

Bend the right ankle and turn the foot up, raising the stretched leg and grasping the toes with the right hand. Remain in the position for a while and lower slowly. Turn on the stomach and stretch with arms over the head. Repeat on the other side. Finally lie on the back and stretch.

Exercise No. 8

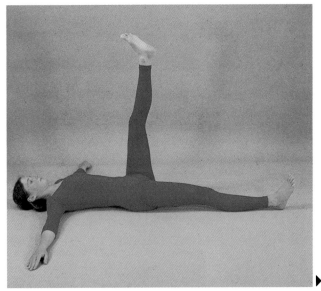

Lie on the back with legs stretched and together, the small of the back on the floor, neck extended. Extend the arms straight out to the sides with palms down. Inhale and raise the left leg to vertical.

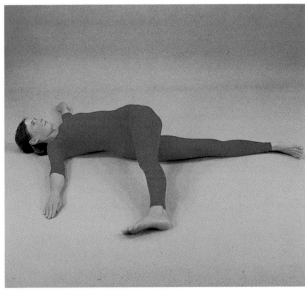

Slowly lower the leg to the right side and exhale, keeping the shoulders on the floor. Inhale, raise the leg to vertical and lower it beside the left one. Exhale.

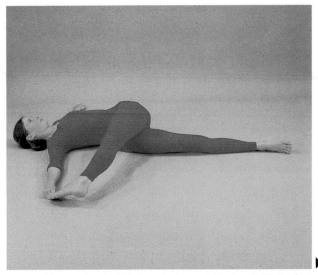

Repeat this exercise, but this time try to reach the hand with the foot when lowering the leg.

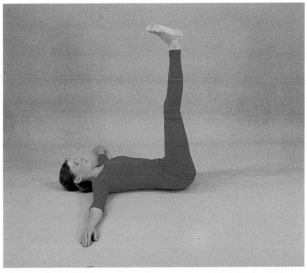

Inhale, pull the abdomen in and press the small of the back down, raising both legs to vertical, and keeping them straight, ankles bent. Exhale and inhale.

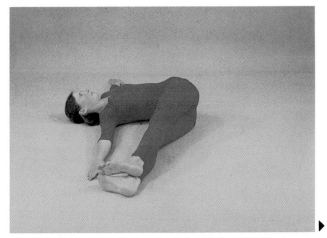

Lower the legs to the right and exhale. Inhale, raise the legs to vertical and lower them straight down, keeping the loins on the floor.

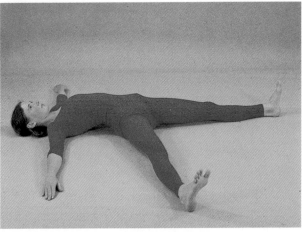

With the feet pointing up, inhale and slide the right leg to the side. Exhale and bring the leg back. Repeat the series with the other leg.

Exercises for the legs and feet

Exercise No. 9

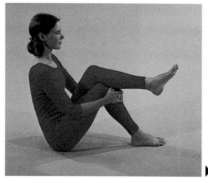

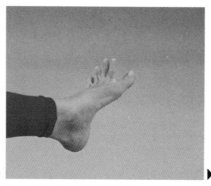

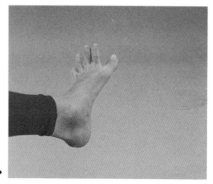

Sit with legs bent. Place the left leg across the right knee and interlock the fingers around the right lower leg.

Spread the toes of the left foot.

Move the big toe upward and downward.

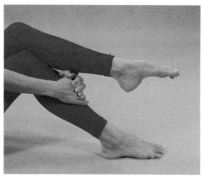

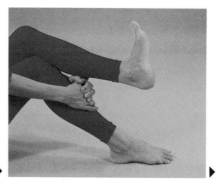

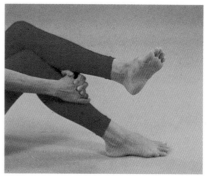

Stretch the ankle and point the toes.

Bend the ankle and point the toes upward.

Rotate the ankle joint a few times in both directions. Relax. Repeat the series with the other foot.

Exercise No. 10

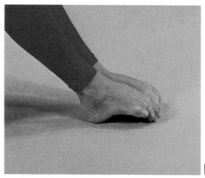

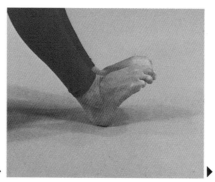

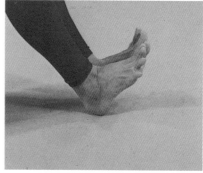

Sit with a straight back and bent legs. Turn your toes under as much as possible.

Resting on the heels, arch the feet as much as possible raising the front part of each foot.

Relax the toes and spread them as far as possible. Lower the feet and repeat a few times.

Exercise No. 11

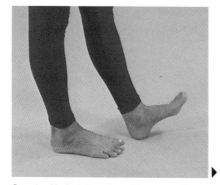

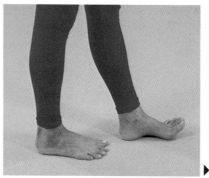

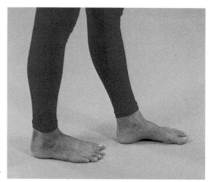

Stand with feet together. Move one foot a little forward, point the toes up and place the heel on the floor ...

lower the metatarsus ...

and lastly the toes. Bring the other foot forward and continue in the same way a few steps.

Exercise No. 12

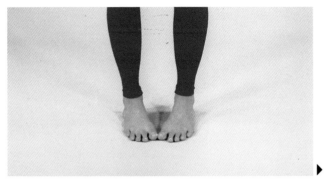

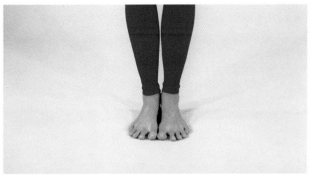

Stand with a straight back, shoulders relaxed. Keep the heels a little apart and the big toes together.

Raise your heels, bring them together and lower, so that the insides of the feet are touching from toes to heels.

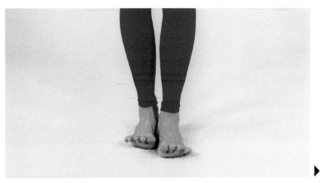

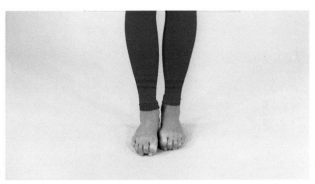

Keeping the shoulders and arms relaxed, pivot on the heels, toes raised, and walk forward with small steps.

Turn your toes under, so that only the toe-tips and heels rest on the floor. Keep the feet from slipping sideways. Walk forward with small steps.

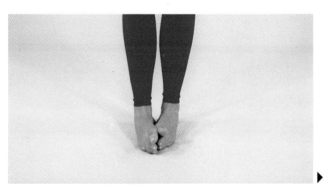

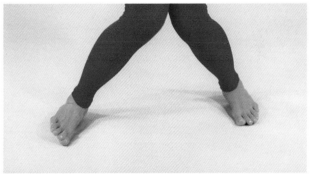

Stand on the outer edge of the feet, so that the soles face each other. Keep the big toes straight and slide your feet forward close to one another.

Place the feet wide apart, so that the heels and the inner edge of the feet rest on the floor. Walk forward with small steps.

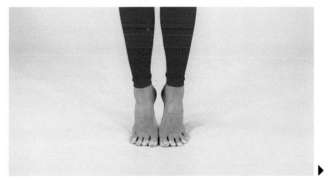

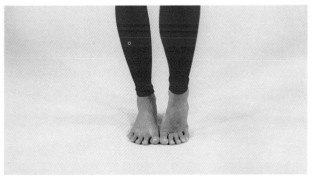

Bring the feet together and spread the toes. Stand up on the toes, stretching the ankles fully. Transfer the weight to the big toes, not allowing the feet to give way at the sides.

Lower the right heel slowly, resting on the toes of the left foot. Rise up on the toes and then lower the left heel. Lower the right and left heel alternately, knees pointing straight forward.

Hand exercises

In general

These exercises improve the conscious co-ordination of muscles, increase the strength and flexibility of the fingers and the wrists, and stimulate the circulation of blood in the hands. Cold hands, rheumatic pains in the hands and forearms as well as inflammation of the synovial sheaths, may all benefit from these exercises.

Exercise No. 1

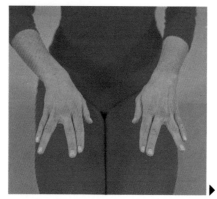

Sit erect with shoulders relaxed and forearms pointing forward. Move the little fingers out to the sides and back, repeat with little and ring fingers together, and with little, ring and middle fingers.

Exercise No. 2

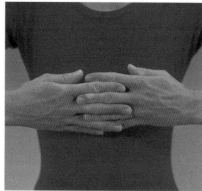

Interlock the fingers with palms toward the body. Slowly pull the hands away from each other with resistance from the pressed fingers. Keep the shoulders relaxed.

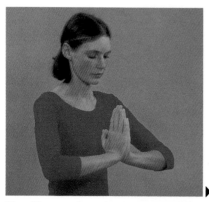

Sit with a straight back and shoulders relaxed. Press the palms together with forearms horizontal.

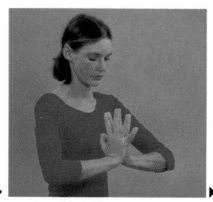

Still pressing the palms together, spread the fingers wide apart. Bring the fingers together and apart several times.

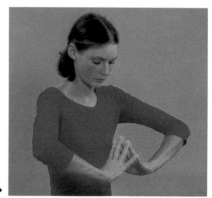

Spread the fingers slightly. Retain the pressure, gradually pulling the palms and fingers apart until only the finger-tips meet. Press backward, slowly bringing the hands together.

Exercise No. 4

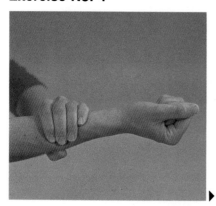

Hold the right forearm with the left hand, keeping the four fingers on top and thumb underneath. Find the muscles used for clenching the fists and stretching the hands.

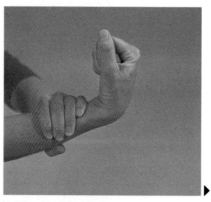

Holding the right arm firmly above the wrist, clench the right hand and bend the wrist up and down several times.

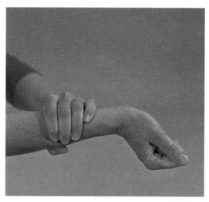

Move the right hand to either side, and rotate in each direction. Repeat the whole exercise with the opposite hand positions.

Chapter 2
Yoga-asanas

This chapter includes 40 classical yoga-asanas and a single combined exercise (suryanamaskar). The technique for the exercises is shown in the form of illustrations of the main stages, with a short instructive text. Some specialised preliminary exercises are shown for the various postures, together with advanced variations.

Most people can begin at once with the practice of yoga-asanas, and children, who usually enjoy the postures, can start at the age of 7 or 8. Elderly people should be particularly careful because of the natural stiffness of their muscles and joints. You should be cautious in case of weakness in the spine, particularly if you have a tendency for slipped discs. If you have any doubt, it is better to consult your doctor before beginning the exercises. Women should not do yoga-asanas during menstruation or after the second month of pregnancy, but may benefit from the relaxation exercises at those times.

You should not do yoga-asanas just after physical and mental strain. Take a rest and calm the system before you start. Wait at least three hours after a meal. Do not practise asanas on a bed, or on an uneven, slanting or loose surface. Use a mat on firm ground or on the floor, so as to make your posture steady. Avoid tight clothes: wear something light and loose-fitting, which does not hamper movements. Jewellery should be removed beforehand, and the asanas done in an environment free of interruptions and disturbance. Do not rush and remember to complete your programme with deep relaxation in savasana.

Name

Sirshasana means head-posture or head-stand, and is considered to be one of the most important asanas.

Effects

The effect of sirshasana are caused mainly by the force of gravitation which works on the body in this posture. The inverted position of the body improves the return flow of venous blood from the legs and abdomen, which are weak parts of the circulatory system. If you stand or sit on a chair for a long time, gravitation will hamper the flow of venous blood from the organs below the heart. This may cause tiredness and painful and swollen legs, and eventually lead to varicose veins. By regular practice of sirshasana these symptoms can be prevented, and in many cases cured. This posture also combats venous stasis in the abdominal cavity, reduces the internal pressure in the pelvis and prevents malfunction and displacement of the abdominal organs. The regulated inter-abdominal pressure improves blood circulation and digestion and makes breathing easier. Sirshasana is also a good exercise to combat piles.

In sirshasana the head and the neck get an ample supply of fresh, oxygenated blood, causing a pleasant and relaxing warmth. This also tones up the facial muscles, skin and sense-organs. In some of the ancient Sanskrit texts, it is said that sirshasana prevents and removes wrinkles. Anyhow, it refreshes and relaxes the face and head and may remove certain kinds of tension and headaches. The posture is an ideal exercise for people who do strenuous mental work. It is known to still the thoughts, sharpen the memory and to increase mental energy. It also prevents sleeplessness and nerve degeneration.

In sirshasana, the expanding upward movement of the ribs is relieved of gravitational pressure, making inhalation effortless and costal breathing the dominating breath. Owing to the pressure on the diaphragm by the abdominal organs, respiration tends to be shallow, but if you consciously attempt diaphragmatic breathing (p. 126), you can easily get a clear conception of muscular activity in deep

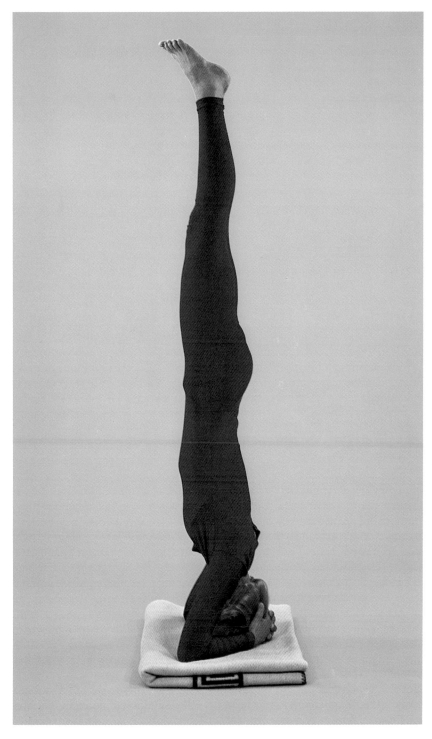

yogic breathing, and its connection with the nerve currents. By the regular practice of sirshasana, you may therefore learn to remove nervous tension in the area of the solar plexus and in the abdominal muscles.

During the initial stages of practice, it is particularly important to be attentive to keeping the balance of the body, and to remain relaxed. This will improve your power of concentration, reduce restlessness and make

it easier to meditate. Yogis who practise mind-control use this asana as a means to convert sexual energy into mental power (ojas shakti), and to awaken the hidden power of consciousness (Kundalini Shakti), which is the key to and substance of higher spiritual development. However, to gain these effects it is necessary to combine the practice of sirshasana with regular and systematic meditation and to regulate diet and lifestyle.

Sirshasana

In general

Sirshasana should be learned with care and caution to prevent any damage to the cervical vertebrae, or the fine blood vessels in the head. Begin by finding the right point of support on the top of the head by standing barefooted, with the heels, back and neck against a wall and with a book on your head. The place on which the book rests in free balance is the point on which you should stay in sirshasana. Next, you should gradually make the body accustomed to the reversed position. It is particularly important that the delicate blood vessels of the head and brain become used to the increased pressure and supply of blood. You should be familiar with the different phases of sirshasana before practising the final posture with legs raised, and be sure that you can tolerate the pressure.

When commencing the posture, place the front of the scalp on a folded blanket. During the entry phase, the point of contact will automatically roll on to the crown, so that the neck is straight. It is important that the hands are folded around the back of the head, acting as a support and not as something to stand on. If you rest the head on the hands, the weight will be more on the frontal part. This causes a skewing effect on the cervical vertebrae, and tension in the neck muscles. When you take up the static phase, you may practise near a wall or have someone close by. These should not be used as supports, but only as safety measures in case you lose your balance. If you fall from the position, you simply double up and roll gently down on your back.

If sirshasana is done correctly, you should be completely motionless and relaxed, while the breath flows in a quiet and easy rhythm. If you are tensed, or there is pain in the neck and shoulders, or if you get jerky contractions and cannot stay still, the posture may be wrong and it should be abandoned. It may be difficult to discover the fault yourself and it is a good idea to let an experienced person check your technique.

During the entry and exit phases you should avoid any sudden jerks, and move the body in a soft, gliding way. In the exit phase, follow the same movements as the entry phase, but in reverse order.

Sirshasana should not be attempted if you have any weakness in the spine, bad arteriosclerosis or a weak heart. The posture should also be avoided in cases of any discharge from the ears, weak eye capillaries or if you have a loose retina. If you want to take up this asana after the age of 50, or if you are receiving medical treatment for high blood pressure, then you should first consult your doctor.

Duration

There are no hard and fast rules for the time you may stay in sirshasana, and there is a large variation depending on the individual capacity and the particular kind of training of which the posture may form a part. Advanced yogis may remain in sirshasana for up to 3 hours at a stretch. People who practise meditation and sex-sublimation (sadhakas) remain in the posture up to a quarter of an hour, but if you practise the asanas purely as a physical exercise, you should limit the time to some seconds in the beginning, gradually prolonging it to 4, or 5, minutes, once a day. At any rate, you should be careful and closely watch the effects and regulate the period accordingly. If you become over-heated or feel pressure in the head, a buzzing in the ears, or get bloodshot eyes, it indicates that you cannot tolerate the posture or have remained in it for too long.

Technique I

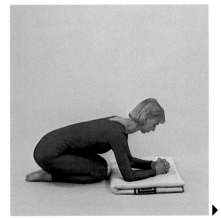

Kneel down and place the forearms on a folded blanket with the elbows apart at shoulder width so the upper arms are vertical. Clasp the fingers together.

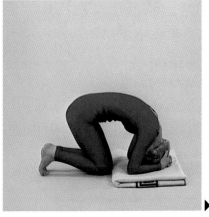

Place the forehead on the blanket between the forearms. Lift the buttocks and roll onto the crown of the head, until the neck is straight and vertical, cupping the back of the head with the hands.

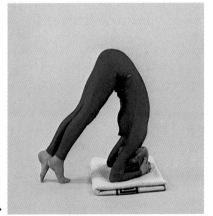

Straighten the legs and walk towards the body, lifting the hips high until the back is straight and the thighs touch the body. Transfer the weight of the body to the head and elbows.

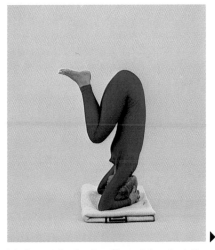

Inhale, retain the breath and bend at the knees. The feet will rise quite effortlessly from the floor if the pose is correct, and the back is strong enough.

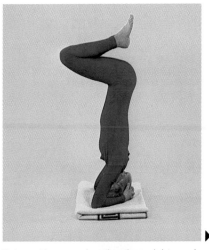

Balance the pose, keeping the weight evenly distributed on the head and elbows, as you raise the thighs to horizontal.

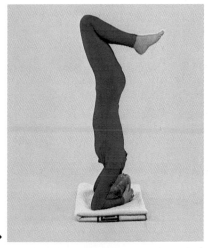

Continue raising the thighs towards vertical, moving the feet backward. Avoid overarching the back.

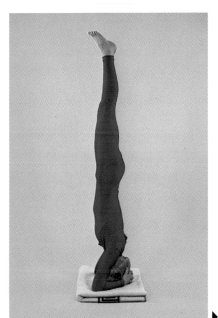

Stretch the legs to vertical and exhale. Align the body by tightening the buttocks and levelling the pelvis as you push the soles of the feet towards the ceiling. Remain in the pose, as relaxed as possible, breathing deeply and regularly.

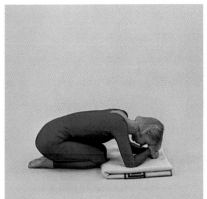

Inhale and quietly return from the pose, following the entry phases in reverse order. Exhale resting on the heels. Place the clenched fists upon each other and rest the forehead on them. Inhale through wide open mouth, retain breath as long as comfortable and exhale slowly through the nose. Repeat twice. Tuck in your chin and roll up to vajrasana (p. 97). Stand up and align the spine, lifting the top of the head and the breast bone, with chin and buttocks slightly tucked in. Raise the arms over the head and stretch well. Relax in savasana (p. 108).

Sirshasana

Technique II

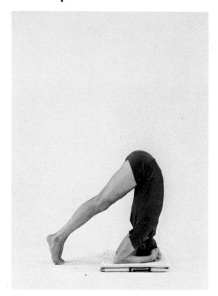 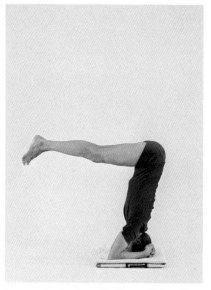 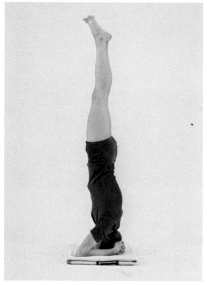

Follow technique I until the back is straight.

Inhale and raise the extended and joined legs to horizontal and higher up in a smooth movement ...

until the whole body is straight and vertical. Exhale and breathe deeply and regularly. Lower the legs and finish as under technique I.

Variations

This series develops the balancing powers, renders the hip joints flexible and exercises the muscles of the legs. The series should only be performed when you have mastered sirshasana and are familiar with its effects. Each pose of the series may be done separately.

1. Follow one of the above-mentioned techniques of sirshasana. Bring the left leg forward and the right leg backward. Repeat to the other side.

2. Try to keep the right leg vertical while lowering the left leg until the foot reaches the floor. Repeat with the other leg.

3. Spread the legs apart as much as possible and tuck in the buttocks so the pose remains straight.

4. Bring the legs into padmasana (p. 112) by placing one instep in the opposite groin and bend the knees a little forward as you move the other foot into a similar position. Point the knees towards the ceiling, aligning the body so it becomes straight. Carefully move the legs out of padmasana, stretch the feet towards the ceiling and come down following technique I or II.

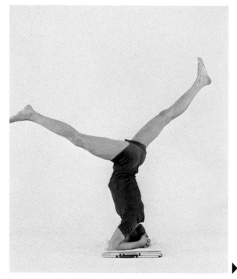 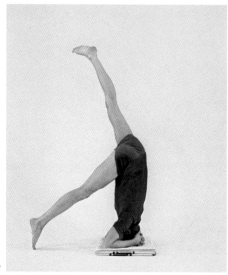

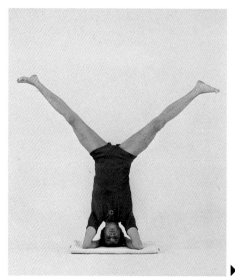 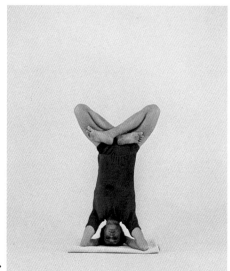

Preliminary exercises

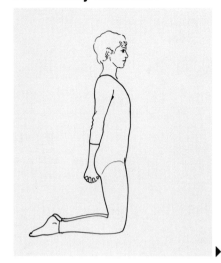

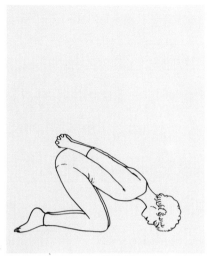

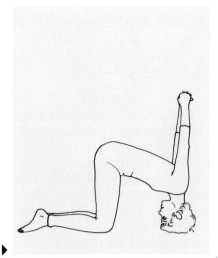

1. Kneel upright and clasp the fingers behind the back, pulling the shoulders downward and together.

Inhale, concaving the spine, and bend forward extending the breast-bone and placing the forehead on the floor. Exhale.

Roll up to rest on the crown of the head so the neck is vertical, and move the arms towards the ceiling. Breathe deeply and regularly in the pose. Lower the arms and rest the buttocks on the heels, forehead on the floor.

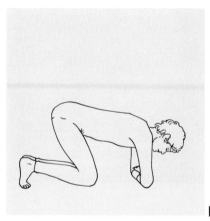

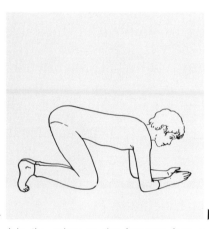

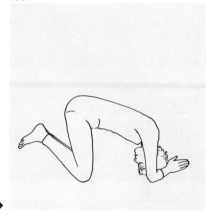

2. Kneel upright and bend forward, placing the elbows on the floor so that the upper arms and thighs are vertical. Measure the distance between the elbows by placing the finger-tips on the opposite elbow.

Join the palms so the forearms form a triangle and place the crown of the head inside this. Make sure the neck is vertical.

Distribute the weight evenly onto the forearms, the top of the head and the knees as you raise the feet from the floor. The feet should remain relaxed. Lower the feet, rest on the heels and relax.

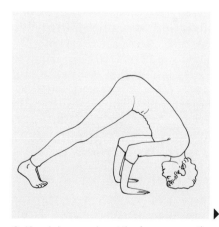

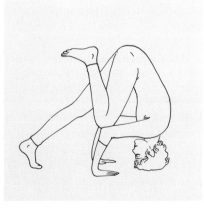

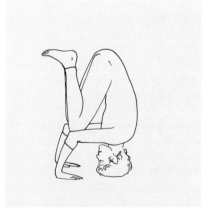

3. Kneel down and rest the forearms on the floor, elbows at shoulder width and fingers together. Place the forehead on the floor between the hands, and put the palms in place of the elbows. Stretch the legs and roll onto the top of the head.

Walk the feet closer to the hands until the back is as straight as possible, and the neck vertical. Place the right knee on the right elbow and bend the lower leg upwards.

Rest the left knee on the left elbow and lift this foot too, when you feel balanced. Relax feet and breathe deeply. Replace the feet and the knees on the floor, sit down on the heels and finish with breaths and a stretch as after sirshasana.

Sarvangasana

Name

Sarvangasana is normally called the shoulder-stand. Sarvanga means "all parts of the body", which indicates the beneficial effects of this posture on the whole system.

Effects

As with sirshasana, the effects of sarvangasana are mainly caused by the force of gravitation, which influences the body inversely when compared with the normal stance. In this posture, there is less pressure on the head and face, and if you find sirshasana difficult then you can try sarvangasana to obtain similar benefit.

The shoulder-stand improves the flow of venous blood from the legs, abdomen and other organs below the heart, thus preventing varicose veins and blood congestion. Sarvangasana tones up the internal abdominal organs, and combats constipation, piles, and enteritis.

When you do sarvangasana, the blood supply to the head, shoulders and neck increases, and all these organs benefit from the improved flow during the relaxation phase. Experiences from regular practice suggest that sarvangasana normalises the function of the thyroid gland and thereby the general metabolism. This effect may be ascribed to the pressure of the chin-lock (jalandhara bandha, p. 120) and the increased flow of blood to the throat area. The posture also reduces muscular tension in this area, producing a relaxating, warm sensation in the chest and head.

The pressure of the chin against the breast-bone hampers costal breathing in sarvangasana, but as the abdominal organs pressure the diaphragm, you can easily feel and understand how to exercise this organ and activate deep abdominal respiration. This makes sarvangasana an ideal exercise for people who breathe superficially.

In sarvangasana you will experience how fatigue, tension and mental depression give way to a sensation of life and lightness flowing through the whole system. This posture also reduces the innumerable aimless thoughts that crowd the mind, making you experience some inner rest or peace which helps to calm your wor-

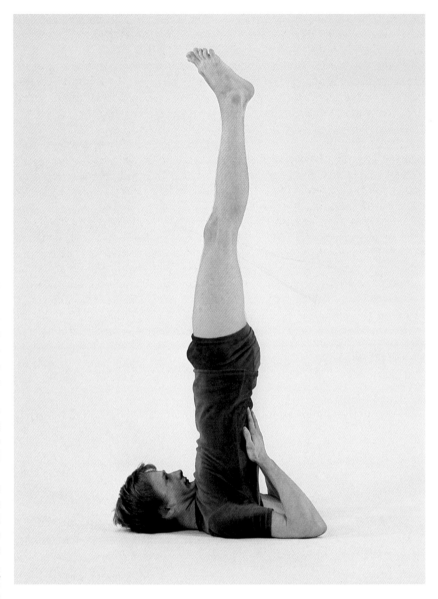

ries, stresses and emotions.

The Indian yogis attribute to sarvangasana rejuvenating powers which help to keep the body vital and youthful. It is also used as a means to sublimate sexual energy, thus leading this enormous power in the direction of superior physical and mental health, together with spiritual awakening.

In general

When you raise your stretched legs from the supine position, it is important to tighten the muscles of the buttocks and the pelvis, to pull the abdomen inward and upward and press the small of the back against the floor; if not, you may increase the pressure in the pelvis and strain the lumbar area, which is a delicate part of the back. If you suffer from prolapse of any organs in the abdominal cavity, weak

abdominal muscles or an excessive lumbar lordosis, you should avoid raising your stretched legs until you have trained yourself, e.g. with abdominal exercises Nos. 2 and 3 (p. 39) and uddiyana bandha (p. 121). Until you have become fit, you can enter sarvangasana by bending your knees towards your chest and then lifting your buttocks and back, pressing your palms onto the floor. With the body resting on the shoulders, and the bent knees just above the face (see preliminary exercise No. 1), move your elbows together as much as possible and support the back with your hands. Lastly, stretch out your legs in a vertical position. The position of the hands is vital for the final posture. Unless the back is supported in the correct place, the body will slant, making the chin-lock imperfect, restraining the abdominal breath and quickly tiring the arms. To get the body into a straight, vertical position, the hands should support the back as close to the shoulder blades as possible. If the posture is done correctly, the chin should be firmly pressed against the breast-bone, and the trunk and legs be in a straight, vertical position, so that the whole weight rests on the shoulders and arms. Do not press the teeth or contract the abdominal muscles or legs, and try to remain motionless in the posture.

In the beginning, the subdued costal breathing may make respiration somewhat strenuous, and there may be some jerky movements in the respiratory muscles. It is therefore important to relax consciously and to concentrate on making the movements of the diaphragm deep and rhythmical.

When you master the posture and relax in it, you should try to concentrate on a certain sensation of well-being that flows through the whole organism from the feet to the head. You may also concentrate on the throat area and imagine that good, healthy and rejuvenating energies are radiating from it and penetrating the whole body.

Come down from the posture by lowering the legs over the face and stretch the arms down behind you. Press the palms of the hands on the floor, and roll the back down little by little. When the loins have been lowered, tighten the pelvic muscles, draw in the abdomen and press the small of the back onto the floor, while lowering the extended legs. Beginners may bend the knees against the chest after lowering the back, and place the feet on the ground next to the buttocks, before stretching out their legs and relaxing.

In case of defective vertebrae in the neck, a weak heart or high blood pressure, you should be very careful. With enlargement of the thyroid you may do preliminary exercise No. 3, to avoid pressure on the throat.

Duration

In the beginning, you should limit the time of sarvangasana to a few seconds, and closely observe the effects during and after the exercise. Gradually increase the time up to 4 or 5 minutes.

Technique

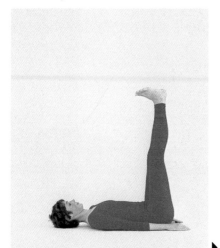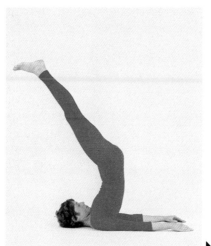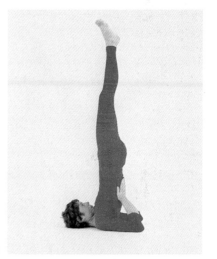

Lie flat on the back, chin in, palms down. Inhale, contract the buttocks, tuck in the stomach and press the small of the back onto the floor, raising the extended legs together.

Press the palms down, lifting the trunk as you bring the legs above the head. Support the back with the palms close to the shoulder blades and exhale.

Straighten the body so it becomes perpendicular, pulling in the buttocks and lifting the breast-bone. Relax as much as possible, breathing deeply in the pose.

Variations

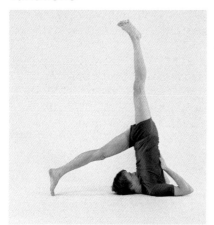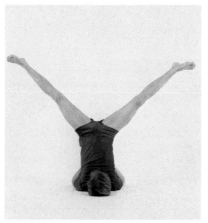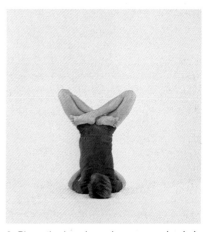

1. Lower the right leg towards the floor behind the head. Repeat with the left leg.

2. Spread the legs as wide apart as possible keeping the buttocks in.

3. Place the legs in padmasana as in sirshasana var. 4 (p. 52). Try to remain straight.

Sarvangasana

Variations

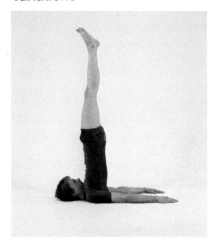

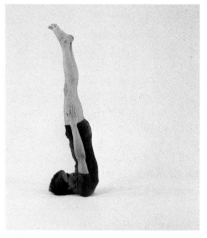

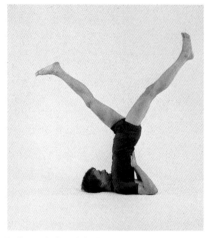

4. Place the arms on the floor behind the back, palms facing down.

5. Extend the arms along the sides of the body, resting on neck and shoulders alone.

6. Stretch the right leg forward, and the left leg equally backward, splitting as much as possible. Repeat on opposite side.

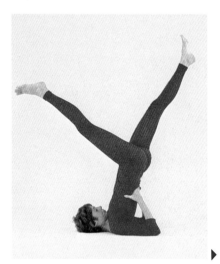

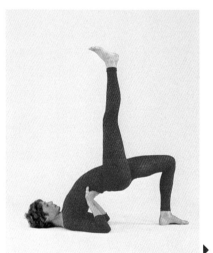

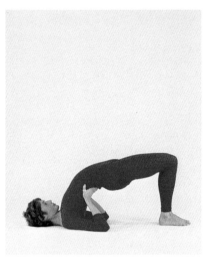

7. Standing in sarvangasana, move one leg forward, slowly lowering the other leg backward.

Bend the posterior leg at the knee and place the foot on the floor. Stretch the upper leg towards the ceiling, with foot relaxed.

Lower this leg too and try to raise the hips further. Extend the arms on the floor and lower the spine carefully, vertebra by vertebra.

Preliminary exercises

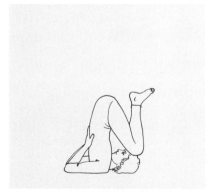

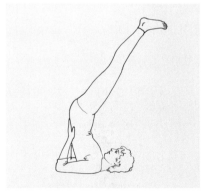

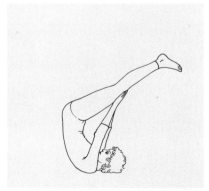

1. Lie on the back, chin in, bend the knees towards the chest and bring them to the forehead lifting the trunk. Place the palms on the back, raising the breast-bone and hips high. Extend the legs over the head and press the palms onto the floor, carefully lowering the back.

2. From preliminary exercise No. 1, you may lift the knees and finally stretch the legs to vertical. Straighten the pose by moving the hands down the back while lifting the breast-bone. Carefully lower the arms and back, then bend the knees towards the chest and rest the feet on the floor.

3. Rest on the upper part of the back and tilt the legs over the head. Place the right hand on the right knee, balance the pose and bring the left hand to the left knee. Arms and legs remain straight. Relax the pose, breathing tranquilly.

56

Name

Viparita karani means reverse action.

Effects

Viparita karani has the same beneficial effects on blood circulation, the abdominal organs, digestion and breathing, as the other inverted postures. There is less pressure on the head and neck than in the two previous asanas, so if these do not suit you they can be replaced by this exercise. The speciality of this posture is its effects on the nervous energies, particularly in controlling the abdominal and pelvic regions. Viparita karani reduces nervousness around the stomach, and tension in the abdominal muscles and diaphragm. Yogis practise this posture as a mudra (seal), that helps to transform or sublimate sexual power to higher mental energy (ojas shakti).

Viparita karani may ease some kinds of headache, combat enteritis and give you a feeling of peace and balance in the system.

In general

In this posture, the major part of the weight rests on the wrists and arms, and it may be necessary to strengthen these, for example with the preliminary exercises of mayurasana (p. 73). The hip-bones should rest in the hollow of the hands, so that the forearms become vertical, with the elbows close together. Try to relax the throat, chest and back, so that the region between the shoulder blades rests on the floor. In viparita karani you should do mula bandha, by slightly contracting the muscles of the anus and perineum, as well as jiva bandha, by pressing the tongue against the palate. In the static phase you can imagine that energy flows from the lower parts of the body towards the head. At the same time draw the abdomen in and up.

Duration

Begin by holding the posture for some 30 seconds, gradually increasing the time to about 5 minutes.

Technique

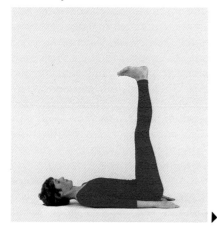

Lie on the back, legs stretched and together, chin in. Inhale and press the small of the back onto the floor, lifting the legs to vertical.

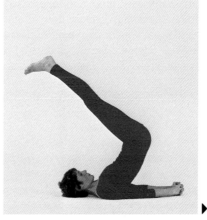

Exhale and raise the back to an angle of 45°. Clasp the fingers and pull backward, bringing the elbows closer. Inhale.

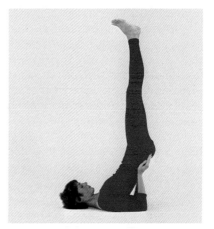

Rest the hips in the palms and exhale. Breathe tranquilly, allowing the breast-bone to sink down. Relax the face, neck and feet.

57

Halasana

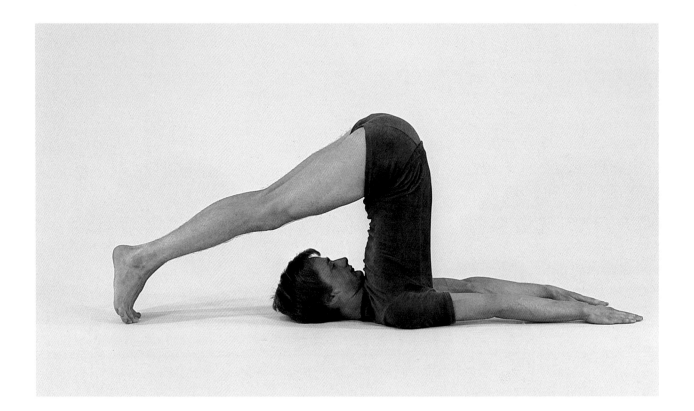

Name

Halasana means plough-posture. It is most probably so named because of its likeness to the ancient Indian bullock-plough.

Effects

Halasana provides an even stretch to the muscles of the back part of the body. It relieves tension in the neck, shoulders and back, toning up these parts and making them supple. The hamstring muscles and buttocks are similarly exercised, which all together render the body alert and flexible. This posture gives you a pleasant warm sensation in the back, as if the nerves themselves are recharged with life and energy, and you are free from tiredness, back pain and headaches. Halasana improves blood circulation in the back, nourishes the cartilages in between the vertebrae, and tones up the nerves of the spinal column through which all the sensory impulses pass. A strong and supple back is vital for our daily well-being and helps to keep the rest of the body in a healthy state. The pressure on the stomach, along with the inverted position, lessens the amount of blood in the abdominal region, causing a suction effect in the relaxed state, thus increasing the passage of blood, which keeps the internal organs healthy. The inverted pose further counteracts descent of the internal organs, and pressure on the stomach improves digestion and releases wind. Regular practice of halasana over a long period of time may normalise irregular menstruation and remove menstrual pain.

In general

Halasana should be done carefully, and prepared for gradually by the aid of some preliminary exercises to avoid over-straining the back. If you find it difficult to touch the floor with the toes, you may bend the legs and rest the knees on the forehead and slowly stretch the legs as much as possible. It relieves strain on the back and may also help to reach the floor if you place the hands against the back, and gently try to press a little to straighten the back vertically. If your back curves too much, you can fold the hands and pull your arms backward, pressing your breast-bone against the chin, at the same time lifting your buttocks high to straighten the spine. If the posture is correct, the weight will rest on the shoulders and neck, and the trunk will be vertical. Respiration should be relaxed.

In halasana the breath is easily strained, especially in people who are overweight, because the abdominal pressure restricts the respiratory movements of the diaphragm. Even the costal breathing is somewhat hampered, and the breath tends to flow in the upper part of the chest. Do not strain respiration unnecessarily by forcing it deeper than it goes by itself; rather concentrate on the respiratory movements of the back. If you are aware of these functions you can adjust your respiration accordingly, breathing lightly and comfortably.

When you master the posture you can increase its effects by gently contracting the muscles of the anus and perineum and drawing in the abdomen. Halasana should not be done if you have any serious problems with the spine, or at least you should first consult your doctor. In case of enlargement of the thyroid, you can do preliminary exercise No. 1, to lessen the pressure on the throat.

Duration

Halasana can be safely done from 1 to 5 minutes once a day, according to your constitution. It may also be done dynamically with three or four short repetitions.

Technique

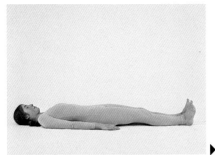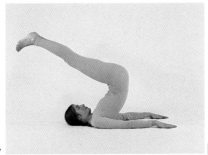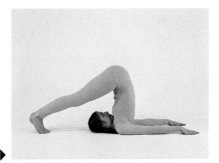

Lie on the back with legs stretched out and together, arms along the sides and palms down. Tuck the chin in, elongating the neck.

Inhale, contract the buttocks, tuck in the abdomen and press the small of the back onto the floor. Raise the legs to vertical, and then further over the head until the feet reach the floor.

Exhale, pull the abdomen backward and contract the anus, lifting the buttocks and breast-bone high so that the back becomes straight. Breathe slowly and regularly.

Variations

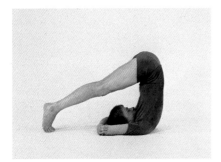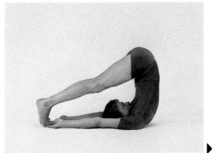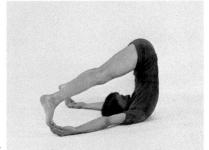

1. Standing in halasana, move the arms around the head and catch hold of the opposite elbow. Concentrate on relaxing the shoulders, as this variation especially removes tensions here.

2. Extend the arms and grasp the toes, sliding the back slightly backward to rest between the shoulder blades.

Pull the legs widely apart. Join the feet again and press the palms onto the floor behind you, before lowering the back.

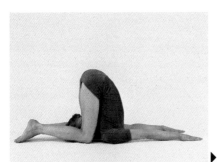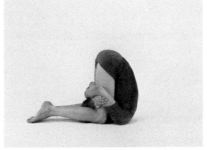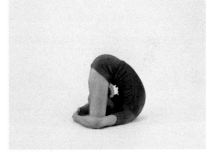

3. Bend the knees and place them on the floor close to the ears, tilting the body toward the chin and keeping the back lifted.

Fold the arms around the hollow of the knees and breathe deeply and regularly.

4. Lie on the back and place the legs in padmasana (p. 112). Inhale and bring the legs over the head until the knees rest on the floor. Place the arms around the knees.

Preliminary exercises

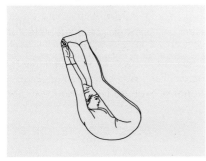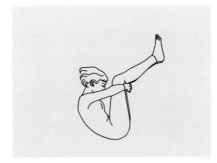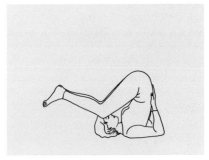

1. Lie flat on the back. Bend the knees towards the chest and raise the legs to vertical. Grasp the feet and pull them over the head until they reach the floor, gently rocking on the upper back.

2. Bend the legs and clasp the fingers around the back of the knees. Lift the head to the knees, pulling the elbows sideways, and rock gently on the back, trying to reach the floor with the feet.

3. Lie on the back, bend the knees to the chest and place them on the forehead, lifting the hips high. Support the back with the hands and lower the feet towards the floor, relaxing them.

Matsyasana

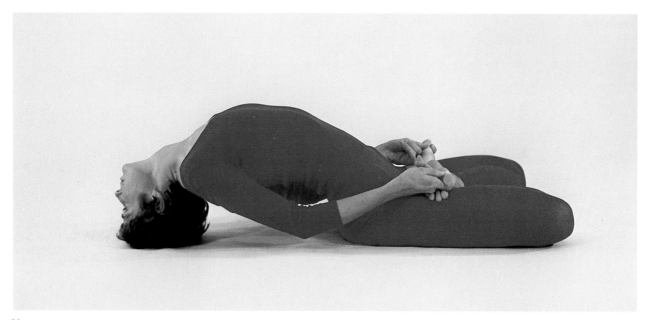

Name

Matsyasana means the fish-posture. Matsya was a mythological fish, who saved humanity from a great flood.

Effects

Matsyasana is naturally connected with both sarvangasana and halasana, because it stretches the front of the body and slightly contracts the back, thereby neutralising any tensions left by the previous postures, so that the physical balance is retained. A combination of these three exercises will keep your spine supple and healthy. The frontal stretch corrects the wrong forward carriage of the shoulders, expands the chest and roots out tension in the chest muscles, thus improving costal breathing, and making you aware of this kind of respiration. Matsyasana is a good exercise for those with asthma and bronchitis. It also relieves nervousness in the solar plexus and tones up the abdominal organs. The muscles of the pelvic region are strengthened and the pain from piles may also be eased. This posture stretches the muscles of the thighs and makes it easy to sit in padmasana (p. 112).

In general

To do the classical matsyasana, you must be able to sit in padmasana, but it can also be done with the legs in other positions. Owing to the stretching of the thigh muscles you may find it hard to get the knees down on the floor. Do not try to force them down, rather be aware of relaxing the muscles of your legs and hips.

In the entry phase you should draw the shoulder blades together before bending the neck backward. In spite of this, some may still get dizzy or have some other unpleasant sensations in the head. In that case it is better to do the variation with the head and neck flat on the floor. The same variation, or preliminary exercises No. 2 and 3 can be done if you have a tendency for slipped discs or suffer from degenerative arthritis in the cervical spine.

Duration

Initially for a few seconds only, increasing gradually up to some minutes. The traditional duration is one-third of the time spent in sarvangasana. If you remain in matsyasana for a longer time, you should do the straight variation.

Technique

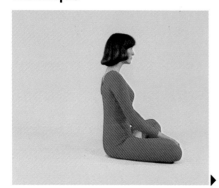

Sit in padmasana (p. 112). Place the palms on the floor beside the hips. Inhale and lean back carefully to rest on the elbows.

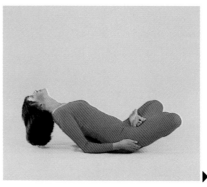

Raise the knees and curve from waist to neck, extending the breast-bone, and place the crown of the head on the floor and exhale. Lower the knees and grasp the big toes.

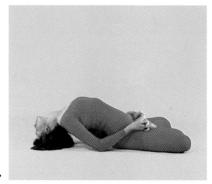

Breathe tranquilly and return to resting on the elbows as you lift the head and knees. Lower the spine, vertebra by vertebra. Unfold the legs carefully and join the knees together before stretching.

Variations

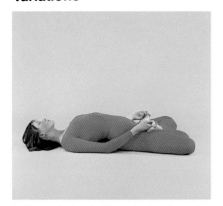 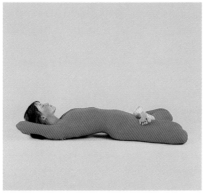 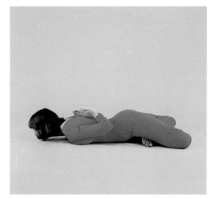

1. Lie on the back. Place the legs in padmasana, lifting the knees. Grasp the big toes and lower the knees onto the floor, relaxing the hip joint and lower back.

2. Lying in var. 1, extend the arms beside the head and cross the forearms, placing the palms under the shoulder blades. Relax and breathe deeply.

3. Sit in padmasana. Reach forward as far as possible and rest on your palms. Roll forward on the knees to lie face down, with chin on the floor. Join the palms between the shoulder blades.

Preliminary exercises

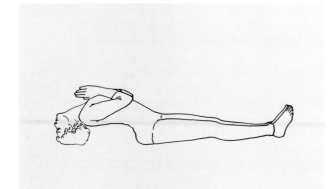 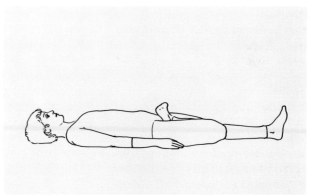

1. Lie on the back, arms along the sides. Inhale, lift the head and upper back, resting on the elbows. Join the shoulder blades together, place the crown of the head on the floor and exhale. Join palms in front of the chest. Rest on the elbows as you raise the head and lower the back, vertebra by vertebra.

2. Lying on the back, bend one knee and carefully place the instep on the opposite thigh, as close to the groin as possible. Relax and allow the knee to sink towards the floor. Repeat with the other leg.

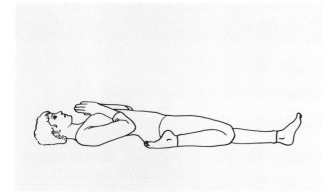 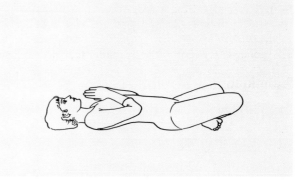

3. Bend the right leg and using the hand place the foot outside the right hip, with the soles facing upward. Try to keep the knee on the floor. Join the palms in front of the chest and relax, breathing deeply. Repeat with the other leg.

4. Lie on the back, bend the knees and cross the legs so that both knees rest on the opposite foot. Relax the lower back, hips and legs. Remain in the pose, breathing deeply, with the palms together in front of the chest, or both arms resting on either side of the head.

Bhujangasana

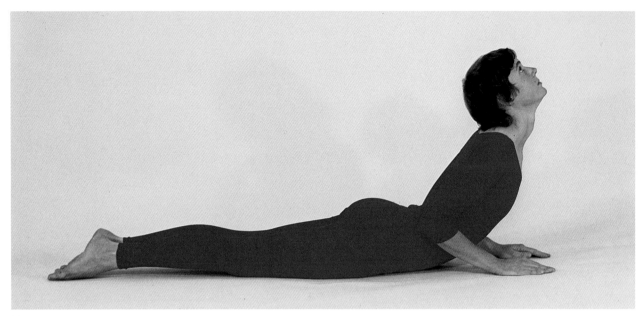

Name

Bhujangasana means the snake-posture. This asana may look like a cobra with raised hood.

Effects

Bhujangasana strengthens the muscles of the back, makes the spine flexible. This exercise is particularly good for the delicate regions of the neck and loins. It may correct minor displacements between the vertebrae, thereby preventing slipped discs and stooping, and relieving tiredness and pain in the back. Bhujangasana stretches the muscles of the chest and prevents weak and drooping shoulders. Though you retain the breath in the posture, it is a kind of breathing exercise that particularly improves the costal breath, and directly exercises and strengthens the heart.

In the relaxing phase you may experience a pleasant warmth in the back, especially in the lumbar region. This may come partly from an increased blood-flow, and also from the increased currents in the spinal nerves, that are vital for the general functioning of the whole system.

Bhujangasana counters constipation and wind, and it is one of the few yoga-asanas which can be done just after a meal.

In general

In this posture the backward bend of the body should begin in between the upper cervical vertebrae and continue downward, vertebra after vertebra, and end with a maximum bend in the lumbar area. It is a common fault to bend the loins initially, and then press the body further back with the arms. Lower the shoulders, draw the shoulder blades together and use the arms as little as possible when you raise the body. Make sure that the legs and buttocks remain relaxed.

Bhujangasana with kumbhaka (retaining the breath) may cause some palpitation in the beginning, as well as an unpleasant pressure in the head. This can be avoided by breathing normally in the pose, which you should also do in case of too high blood pressure.

If you have any defects in the cervical vertebrae or if you easily feel giddy, do not bend the head backward, but keep the neck straight and the chin slightly drawn in against the throat.

Duration

Bhujangasana can be done 2 or 3 times, with a short rest in between. Remain in the posture for as long as you can comfortably hold the breath. If you breathe in the static phase you can keep the pose for about a minute.

Technique

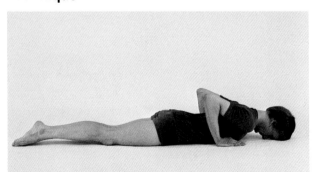

Lie face down with legs together and toes pointing, forehead touching the floor and palms resting on either side of the chest. Keep the shoulders back and arms close to the trunk so that the shoulder blades are together.

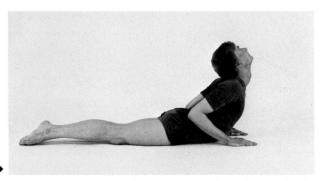

Inhale and curve the back from the neck to the waist, vertebra by vertebra, using the muscles of the back. Only lift to the navel. Come down slowly by relaxing from the waist to the neck and place the forehead on the floor. Exhale.

62

Variations

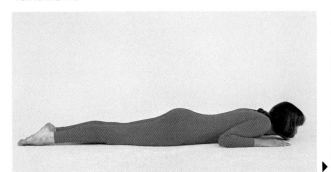

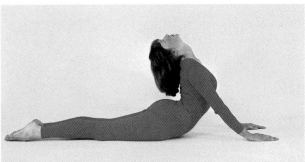

1. Lie face down, chin on the floor and legs together. Place the forearms on the floor, elbows close to the trunk, hands by the shoulders.

Lift the head and curve the back, vertebra by vertebra, extending the breast-bone and pulling the shoulders back and down. Stretch the arms as far as possible, keeping the hips on the floor.

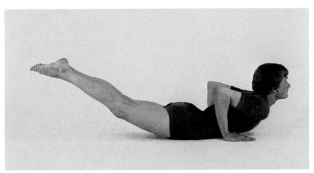

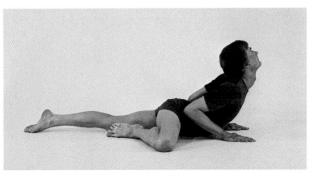

2. Perform bhujangasana and exhale without lowering the trunk. Inhale and raise the extended right leg. Lower leg and trunk and exhale. Repeat with the other leg, and with both legs.

3. Lie face down with the right thigh at right angles to the trunk, and the sole of the right foot against the extended left leg. Perform bhujangasana. Repeat with the left leg bent.

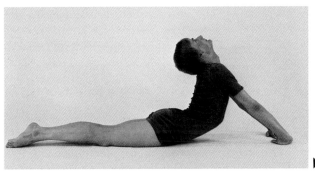

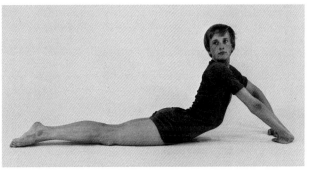

4. Place the palms on the floor under the chin, with the finger-tips touching each other and the elbows facing to either side. Inhale and lift the head and the back slowly. Stretch the arms and exhale.

Inhale, elongating the neck with the chin held in. Bend the left elbow slightly, turning the face to the right shoulder and exhale. Turn to the front, inhale and repeat to the left side. Turn to the front, inhale and lower slowly. Exhale with the forehead on the floor.

Preliminary exercises

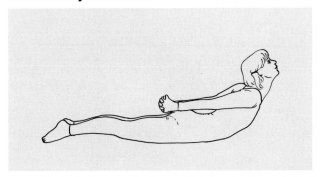

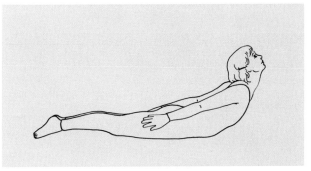

1. Lie with the forehead on the floor and interlace the fingers behind the buttocks. Join the shoulder blades together by pulling the hands towards the feet, and curve from neck to waist. The arms may be lifted in the pose. Come down by relaxing from waist to neck.

2. Commence as in previous exercise, but with the arms alongside the body, and the palms on the thighs. Lift the trunk from the neck to the waist, using the muscles of the back, and come down smoothly. Breathe normally.

Salabhasana

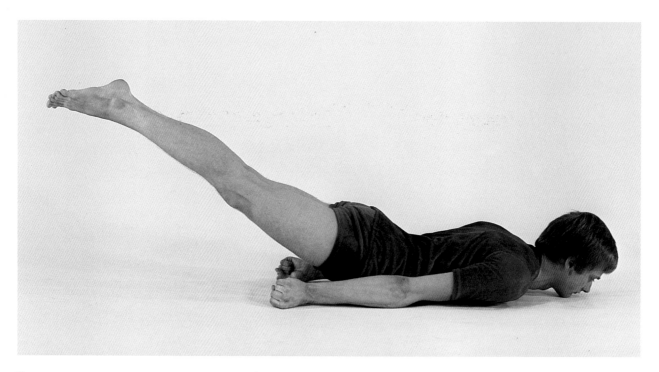

Name

Salabhasana means the locust-posture. The exercise may look like a grasshopper with its raised back.

Effects

Salabhasana is a powerful strengthening and contractive exercise that exercises the muscles of the buttocks, the loins and the back, and to some extent the pelvic muscles also. It improves digestion and may ease some kinds of lumbar and stomach pains. The strong muscular exertion creates a pressure in the abdomen and the head, which spreads to the heart and lungs. Together with the retained breath, and the increased demand for oxygen in the working tissues, this static exercise makes the body vital and alert. As such,

salabhasana also strengthens the lungs and heart muscles and improves the metabolic absorption of oxygen in the body. Salabhasana tones up the nerves of the lower back and strengthens the lumbar muscles in particular.

In general

This asana can be carried out either by stiffening the body before entry or by keeping it as relaxed as possible. In the first method the legs are raised to a higher position, and the internal pressure is rather high, while in the relaxed variation the strain is less and the benefit reduced. In both cases it is the muscles of the lower back that do the main work, while the arms act as support. If you find it difficult to raise both the legs, you can raise one at a

time, or you can place your hands or a rolled-up towel under the upper part of your thighs. The chin and shoulders should remain on the floor.

If you repeat salabhasana, make sure that breathing returns to normal in between each pose. In case of high blood pressure, you should do the exercise in a relaxed manner and breathe normally all the time. Heart patients should not do salabhasana, but may benefit from preliminary exercise No. 1 instead.

Duration

Remain in the posture for as long as it is comfortable to hold the breath. Repeat a few times.

Technique

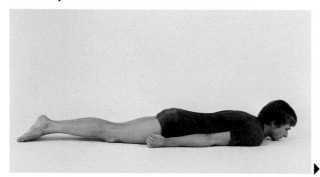

Lie on the stomach, chin on the floor, legs stretched and close together, arms extended along the sides of the body, fists clenched with thumbs down.

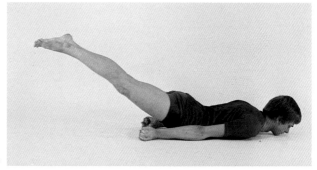

Inhale and extend the legs backward, tighten the buttocks raising legs and hips as high as possible. Keep the knees straight with shoulders and ankles relaxed. Lower the legs quietly and exhale.

Variations

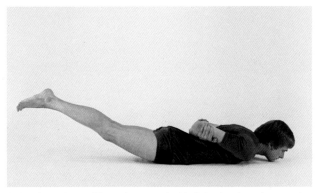

1. Lie face down. Place the arms behind the back and grasp the opposite elbows with the hands. Raise the legs as described.

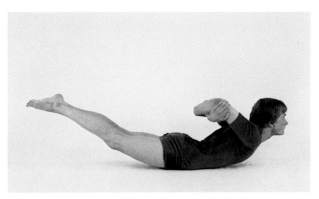

2. Take up the starting position as in var. No. 1. Inhale and raise the legs, head and back simultaneously, pulling the arms backward and upward. Lower arms, forehead and legs, and exhale.

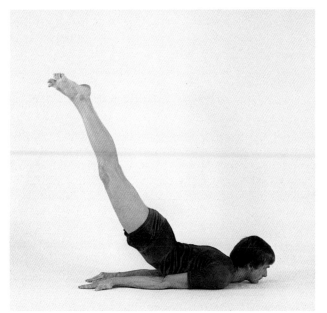

3. By performing salabhasana with arms extended underneath the trunk, pressing the palms of the hands on the floor, it is possible to lift the legs and hips higher.

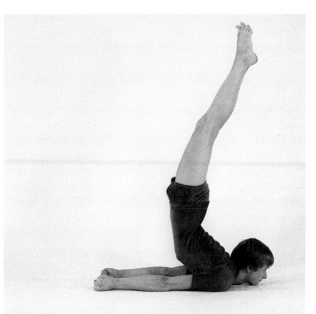

4. This advanced variation is performed with the arms close together, clenched fists, thumbs down. The whole weight is resting on the arms, chest and chin.

Preliminary exercises

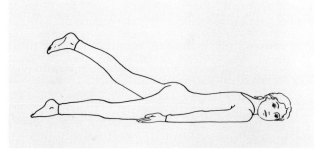

1. Lie on the stomach with the left cheek on the floor, and arms extended close to the trunk. Relax the right side, inhale and raise the left leg straight upward without lifting the hip. Keep the knee straight and the foot relaxed. Lower and exhale. Repeat with the right leg, keeping the right cheek on the floor.

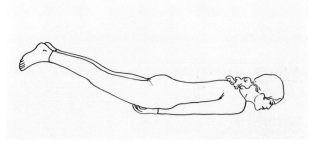

2. Lie with the chin, mouth and nose on the floor, arms underneath the body, palms against the thighs. Extend the legs backward while tightening the buttocks and lifting the legs. Support the thighs with the hands, keeping the knees stretched and together, ankles relaxed. Breathe normally in the initial stage of practice.

Dhanurasana

Name

Dhanurasana means bow-pose. In this exercise the body is tightened up like a bent bow.

Effects

Dhanurasana is a kind of combination of the two previous asanas (bhujangasana and salabhasana), and it is normally done after these asanas. Dhanurasana provides a stretch of the frontal parts, expands the chest, removes tension and stiffness in the shoulders and strengthens the arms and legs. This asana also exercises the lumbar region and may remove pain from the area. If you spend too much time behind a desk or driving, this exercise counters the stooped-forward posture. Dhanurasana stimulates the heart and blood circulation, tones up the nerves of the back, and gives a deep massage to the internal organs. The pressure on and stretch of the abdominal area also decreases nervous tension of the solar plexus.

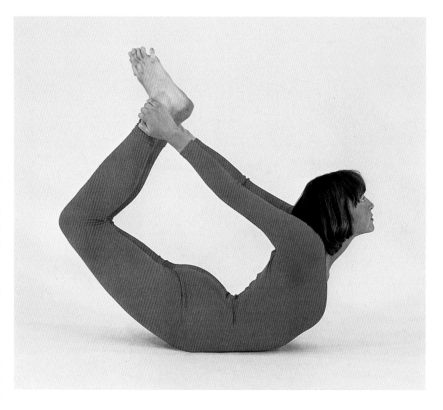

In general

The intensity of dhanurasana depends on the raising of the arms and legs. In the beginning you should be content with a moderate lift and closely observe the character of the exercise and its effects. Be aware of the muscles which are involved in raising the extremities, and those being stretched. Initially it may help your performance to spread the knees, but, if possible, the feet should remain together to make sure that the lift of the shoulders and back is done symmetrically. Try to raise the legs and upper trunk equally, so you rest on your navel, to get maximum benefit. If you get palpitations or feel an unpleasant pressure in the head, you can breathe normally in the posture. If this does not remove the pressure, you can try to bend the head forward a little during the asana. Be careful if you suffer from gastric ulcer or hernia, and use preliminary exercises Nos. 1 and 2 instead.

Duration

Keep the pose for as long as you can hold the breath and repeat a few times without getting exhausted. If you breathe in the posture, be careful not to strain the arms and legs, and limit the time to 1 minute.

Technique

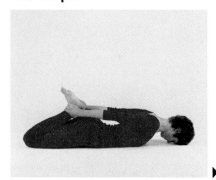

Lie on the stomach with the forehead on the floor. Bend the legs and grasp both ankles, keeping the arms stretched. Turn the soles of the feet toward the ceiling.

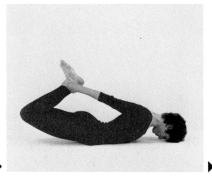

Bring both legs together. Inhale and lift the feet as high as possible, contracting the muscles of the buttocks, while arching in the lower back. Extend the breast-bone.

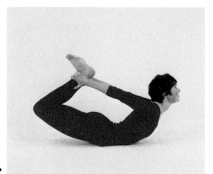

Bend the head backward and push feet and hands higher, keeping the weight of the body on the navel-area. Come down quietly. Exhale with the forehead on the floor.

Variations

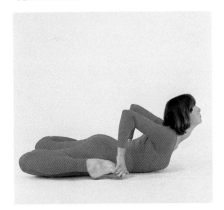

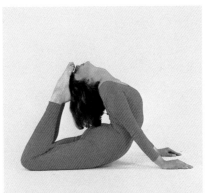

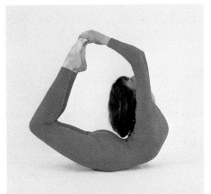

1. Lie on the stomach, chin on the floor. Bend the knees, grasp the feet and cautiously move both feet alongside the hips towards the floor. Pull the elbows together and upward, extend the breast-bone and raise head and upper back, using the muscles of the back and arms.

2. Lie flat with the forehead on the floor, palms down beside the chest and lower legs vertical. Inhale, extend breast-bone and arch backward, stretching the arms. Exhale, bringing the feet and head together. Breathe quietly in the pose.

3. Perform var. No. 2. Exhale, raising the right arm to grasp the right foot, then grasp the left foot with the left hand. Breathe calmly. Push feet and hands upward while exhaling. Lower the knees, bending at the elbows, and place one hand at a time on the floor. Carefully lower forehead and feet.

Preliminary exercises

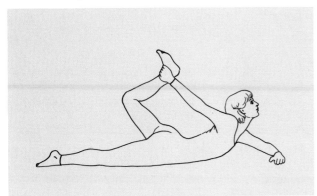

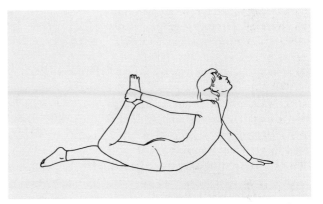

1. Lie on the stomach, the left forearm under the forehead. Bend the left leg and grasp the ankle with the right hand. Inhale and pull the leg straight up without lifting the hip, and bend the head backward. Lower forehead and leg, exhale and relax. Repeat to the other side.

2. Lie face down with the left arm straight forward, palm down. Bend the right leg and grasp the foot with the right hand. Inhale and pull the leg straight up without lifting the hip, and arch backward. Lower quietly and exhale with the forehead on the floor. Repeat with the other leg and arm.

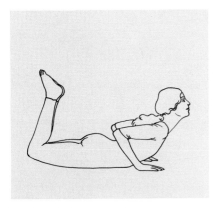

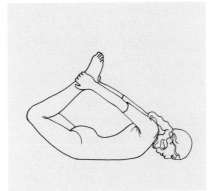

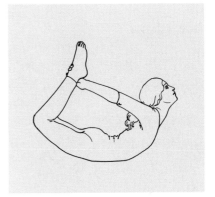

3. Lie with the forehead on the floor, palms down beside the chest and lower legs vertical. Draw the shoulders backward, extend the breast-bone and bend back from the neck toward the waist, using the muscles of the back.

4. Perform dhanurasana, lifting the legs high, keeping the knees apart and the forehead on the floor. Let the breathing be normal and quiet during the initial training.

5. Dhanurasana can be performed with the legs apart, grasping the ankles from the inner side. Breathe normally or retain breath in the pose.

Ardha matsyendrasana

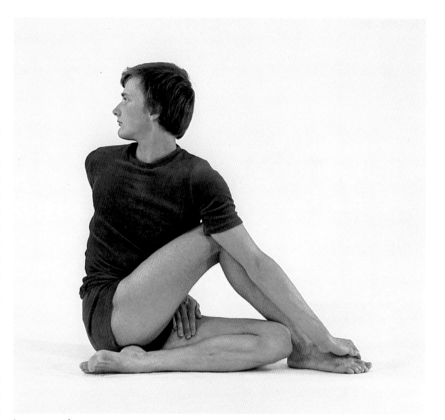

Name

This asana has been named after Matsyendra, who was one of the great masters of hatha yoga. *Ardha* means half.

Effects

Ardha matsyendrasana is one of the few asanas that makes the back supple in an upright position. This effect comes from the rotation of the whole spinal column from the loins to the head. The vertical twist counteracts stiffening and degeneration of the vertebrae. When the flexibility of the spine is attained, and exercises are done regularly, the central nervous system in the spine and its innumerable sensory, motor and visceral impulses will function freely and keep the whole system freshly toned.

Ardha matsyendrasana improves respiration. It expands the chest on one side and gives an upward pressure on the other, which has a cleansing effect on the lungs and makes the respiratory muscles flexible.

In this posture, the muscles on one side are stretched, while there is contraction or pressure on the other side. This alternation creates a kind of suction-and-pump effect on the circulatory system, improving the flow of blood.

The alternate twists of the body also give a deep-reaching massage to all the organs in the abdominal cavity, thereby strengthening them, improving digestion and purifying the blood.

In general

In this asana you should take care to remain seated on both buttocks and keep the body vertically straight, making sure that the knee of the lower leg is kept on the floor. Both the shoulders should be on the same level and should not be raised.

The heel of the lower leg should be placed against the body, but it must not press against the anus, nor should you sit on it. Ardha matsyendrasana should always be repeated on both sides, because the alternate stretching, contraction and pressure are vital to give force and balance to the effects.

If you find it difficult to do the asanas with the lungs inflated, you can breathe out during the entry phase, and hold the breath, or breathe normally in the static phase.

Duration

This exercise is usually done a few times on each side, with retention of breath in the static phase. If you breathe in the posture, limit yourself to one or two breaths.

Technique

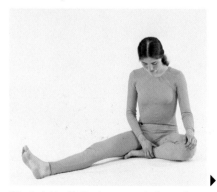

Sit straight with the legs apart in front of you. Bend the left knee and place the foot on the floor close to the groin.

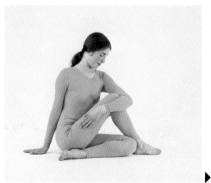

Place the right foot outside the left knee. Bring the left arm round the right knee and push this toward the left armpit. Keep the shoulders level, straighten the back, pulling the trunk toward the right thigh.

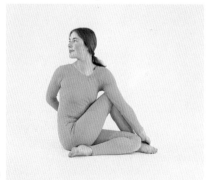

Place the left arm along the outer side of the right leg and grasp the foot. Move the right arm round the back, pulling the shoulder backward. Inhale, stretch the spine and turn to the right from waist to neck. Exhale. Turn forward and repeat on opposite side.

Variations

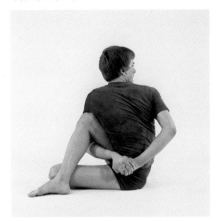 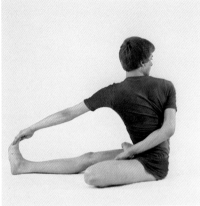 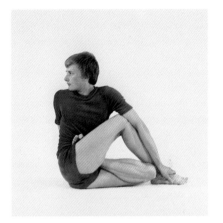

1. Place the legs as described. Bend the left arm under the hollow of the right knee and move it behind the back to grasp the right hand. Inhale, elongating the spine. Turn the head over the right shoulder and exhale. Breathe quietly. Repeat on opposite side.

2. Sit erect with the feet a hip width apart. Place the left instep in the right groin. Grasp the right foot with the left hand, bring the right arm round the back to grasp the left ankle. Inhale, turn to the right, looking over the shoulder, and exhale. Repeat to opposite side.

3. Sit up straight, bend the right leg and place the foot in the left groin. Place the left foot outside the right knee and continue as described under technique. This is the complete pose, matsyendrasana.

Preliminary exercises

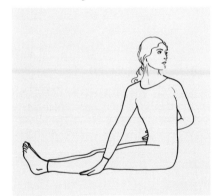 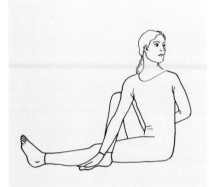 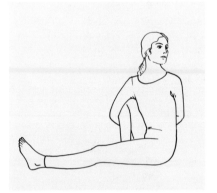

1. Sit erect with the legs apart at hip width. Bring the left arm round the back and place the right hand beside the left knee. Stretch the spine, inhaling. Turn to the left from the hips upward, thereby moving the left foot backward, and the right one forward. Pull the left shoulder backward, look over the shoulder and exhale. Repeat to the right.

2. Sit straight. Place the right foot outside the left stretched knee. Place the right arm along the outer side of the left leg and grasp the right ankle. Move the left arm behind the back. Straighten the spine, inhaling. Turn to the left and exhale. Repeat on the other side.

3. Place the right foot on the floor close to the buttock. Bend the right arm round the knee from the inner side outward. Straighten the spine and twist to the left, moving the left hand round the back to clasp the right hand. Look over the left shoulder. Repeat on the right side.

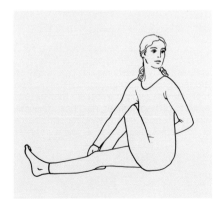 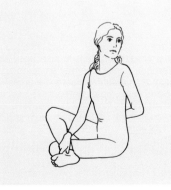 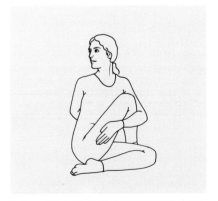

4. Place the left foot outside the stretched right knee. Place the right arm along the outer side of the left leg and grasp the left foot. Move the left arm behind the back. Inhale, extend the spine and turn to the left. Look over the shoulder and exhale. Repeat opposite.

5. Place the right foot outside the left knee and bring the left foot close to the right hip. Grasp the right foot with the right hand and move the left arm round the back. Inhale, extend the trunk and turn to the left until the chin is over the shoulder. Repeat on opposite side.

6. Place the legs as shown under technique. Bend the left arm around the right knee, palm against the thigh. Straighten up the trunk towards the leg. Place the right arm behind the back, twisting to the right from waist to neck. Repeat on opposite side.

Paschimottanasana

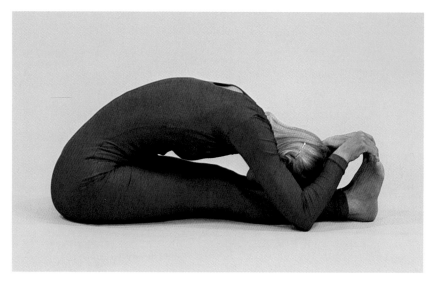

Name

Paschima means back part, and *tan* means stretch. In this posture, the back part of the whole body is stretched.

Effects

As the name suggests, this asana stretches all the major muscles of the back, and the backs of the legs. It makes the back supple, removes pain in the loins and tension in the upper back. Paschimottanasana directly stimulates the energies of the body, removing fatigue and heaviness. It improves the flow of nerve currents all over the back, thereby easing any mental stress and strain which are reflected in these muscles. Regular practice will greatly reduce mental nervousness and nervous disorders all over the body, and make you calm and alert. In India this posture is also called brahmacharyasana, because it helps to sublimate and transform sexual energy into mental power. To achieve this, it is necessary to regulate sexual activity and practise regular meditation.

In general

Because of shortened hamstring and back muscles, it is usually necessary to practise preliminary exercises before one can do the full pose. Sit in the starting position with a slight lumbar sway and try to keep the loins straight, so that the forward bend hinges on the hip joints. This is done by extending the spine, pushing the pelvic region up and forward, and stretching out the chest and chin. If you tend to bend in the loins, it may help to sit on a folded towel, placed right behind your pelvic bones, thus raising and tipping the pelvis a little and making the lumbar region straight. Do not use the arms to drag the body down, as the forward bend should be done by the body itself.

If you find it difficult to reach the feet with the hands, you can grasp your knees, calves or ankles instead.

In this posture, breathe out before beginning the forward bend. During the entry-phase contract the anus and perineum (mula bandha) and draw the abdomen in and up. You can retain the breath during the static phase and again inhale during the exit phase.

If you have trouble with the discs of the lumbar vertebrae, you should do only preliminary exercise No. 3, or some similar exercise in which you can keep the back completely straight.

Duration

If you do paschimottanasana with retained breath, it can be repeated up to about ten times, taking one or two breaths between bends. With normal breathing, paschimottanasana can be done for up to 3 minutes. If you remain longer, it may cause constipation or other abdominal troubles.

Technique

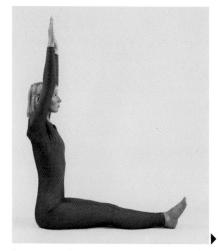

Commence like this: Sit erect with legs together. Inhale raising the arms above the head, elongate and concave the spine. Exhale pulling the abdomen in and up, and bend forward at the hip joint to grasp the toes.

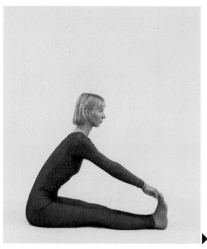

Or like this: Sit erect, the legs together and stretched. Inhale, stretch the spine, extending the breast-bone and grasp the toes. Exhale, pulling the abdomen in and up. Bend forward at the hip joint.

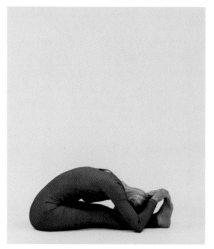

Retain a stretch in the spine as you lower the trunk and face toward the legs. Allow the elbows to sink towards the floor and relax. Keep back and legs as straight as possible.

Variations

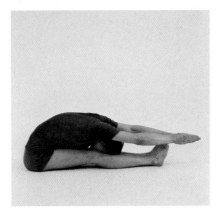

1. Perform paschimottanasana as described and extend the arms as far as possible, just above the feet, thereby increasing the stretch of the back.

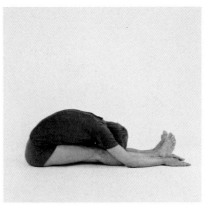

2. Perform paschimottanasana, place the hands and forearms on the floor on either side of the legs and let the arms slide forward as far as possible.

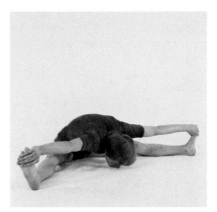

3. Sit straight, legs wide apart, toes pointing upwards. Exhale, drawing the abdomen in, and bend straight forward whilst extending the breast-bone. Grasp the toes and place chin or forehead on the floor.

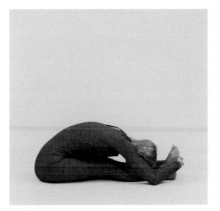

4. Perform paschimottanasana and clasp the hands around the soles of the feet. If possible, stretch the back further over the legs.

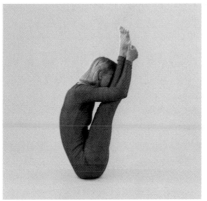

5. Sit up straight with bent legs, feet on the floor close to buttocks. Hold the heels and straighten up one leg at a time. Extend the back and exhale, pulling the trunk toward the legs.

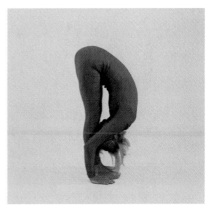

6. Stand erect. Raise the arms above the head inhaling. Extend the spine and sway slightly. Bend forward at the hip joint and exhale, pulling in the abdomen. Place the palms on the floor, or grasp toes or ankles.

Preliminary exercises

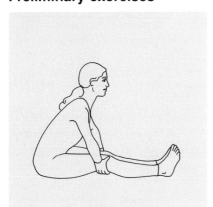

1. Sit erect, legs together and stretched forward. Hold the knees. Inhale and stretch the torso, extending the breast-bone, shoulders back. Exhale, drawing the abdomen in. Bend forward from the hip-joint, pulling the elbows to the sides. Breathe calmly, retaining a steady stretch. Knees and back should remain straight.

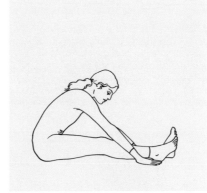

2. Place the palms on the floor on either side of the knees. Walk backward by alternately lifting the right and left buttocks, hands remaining in the same position. Keep the back as straight as possible.

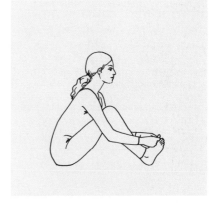

3. Bend at the knees, and grasp the toes with both hands. Keep thighs and trunk close to each other. Stretch the spine and keep the breast-bone and chin raised as you slide the heels forward as far as possible without creating any gap between trunk and thighs.

Mayurasana

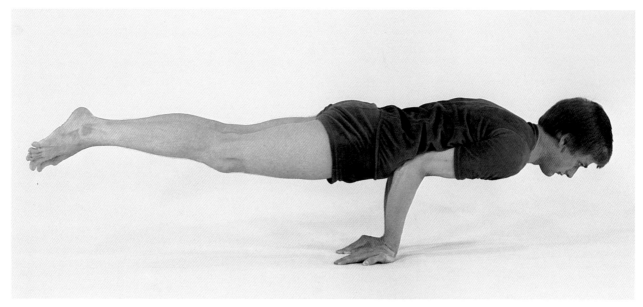

Name

Mayurasana is named after the peacock, owing to its similarity to the long tail feathers of the bird.

Effect

Mayurasana is a very effective balancing exercise requiring a great deal of muscular strength. In particular, the posture strengthens the wrists, and the muscles of the arms, loins, buttocks and abdomen. The powerful pressure of the arms towards the abdominal wall increases the inner pressure in the abdominal cavity; it has a massaging effect on the internal organs in the area, and may help to remove tension around the diaphragm. The posture strengthens the heart and lungs and has a stimulating effect on the function of the abdominal organs; it improves digestion and the function of the intestines, and increases the ability of the organism to remove waste products. Mayurasana is often mentioned in the literature as a good exercise to alleviate diabetes, as the pressure is particularly concentrated in the area of the pancreas. It also has an activating effect on the energies of the body and mind, so that you feel fresh and full of energy. The posture exercises the heart and sends waves of heat through the whole organism, as well as giving a feeling of well-being during the relaxation phase after the exercise.

In general

Mayurasana requires strong wrists and hands, and it is often necessary to do preliminary strengthening exercises. The back muscles may be developed through bhujangasana (p. 62) and salabhasana (p. 64). Begin with the first two phases of the technique, and when the back is sufficiently strong and you are accustomed to the pressure on the abdomen, you can assume the final pose. Owing to pressure in the abdominal cavity breathing is forced, so you may profitably hold the breath after an inhalation.

Mayurasana should not be done when there are wounds in the stomach or intestines, hernia or organic heart disease.

Duration

Begin with a couple of seconds and gradually increase the time up to about 1 minute, or so long as it is comfortable. If pains, violent heart palpitations or shaking arise, then you have exceeded your capacity.

Technique

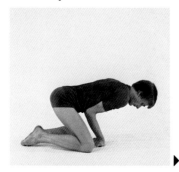 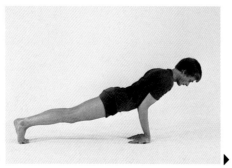 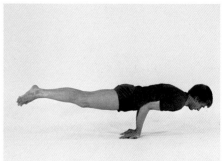

Sit in vajrasana (p. 97) with the knees apart. Place the hands on the floor between the knees, fingers pointing backward. Lift the buttocks and transfer the weight of the body to the forearms, pressing the elbows against the area of the navel.

In this phase beginners may rest the forehead on the floor. Stretch one leg at a time backward so that the body is resting on the bent toes and the hands.

Lean forward a little further, inhale and raise the legs and head from the floor, keeping the body straight and firm in the pose. Exhale, lowering legs and trunk slowly.

Variations

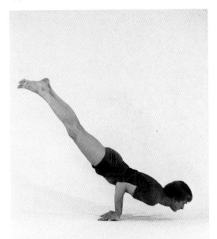

1. Lower the upper body slightly, lifting the legs higher.

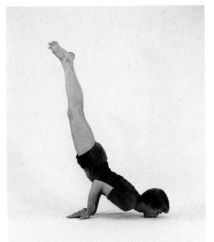

2. Rest the chin on the floor, contract the buttocks and raise the legs as far as possible towards the ceiling.

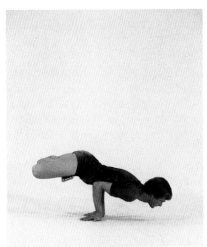

3. Place the legs in padmasana (p. 112), rest on the knees and perform mayurasana as described under technique.

Preliminary exercises

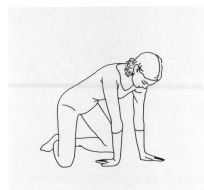

Kneel down with knees apart and feet together. Rest the left hand on the floor, fingers outward, and the right hand between the knees, fingers pointing toward the toes.

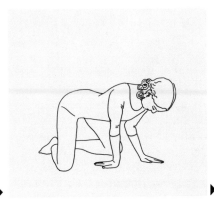

Bend the right elbow toward the navel, lean forward and transfer the weight of the body to the right arm.

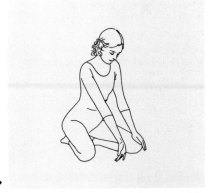

Slowly lean back to sit on the heels, while gradually lifting the right palm from the floor, the three middle finger-tips staying on the floor. Repeat with the opposite arm position.

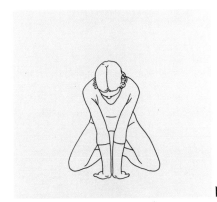

Place both palms beside each other on the floor between the knees, fingers pointing toward the feet.

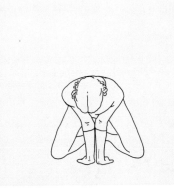

Bend the arms, so the elbows are together, pressing against the area of the navel. Remain in the pose for a while, transferring the weight of the body to the hands.

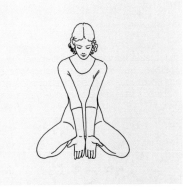

Slowly lower the buttocks to rest on the heels, gradually raising both palms off the floor, without lifting the finger-tips of the middle fingers. Repeat a few times.

Supta Vajrasana

Name

Supta means lying and *vajra* is the thunderbolt of the god Indra.

Effect

Supta vajrasana can be used when matsyasana (p. 60) is too difficult. Supta vajrasana stretches the front part of the body and removes tension in the respiratory and abdominal muscles. The chest is lifted and expanded so that breathing becomes easy, and the posture is well known for its curative effect on diseases of the respiratory system. The stretching of the abdomen has a stimulating effect on the internal organs and counteracts constipation. The posture helps to control nervous activity in the solar plexus, which in the case of stress can cause static tension in the respiratory and abdominal muscles. It is an excellent remedy for a nervous stomach. People engaged in sedentary work, who sit in a bent posture at their desks, would be well advised to do this posture a couple of times during the course of the day. It recharges the vital energy, facilitates mental activity, removes pain in the neck and loins and gives a feeling of lightness to the whole body. In the long term it helps to prevent wearing down and degeneration of the spinal column.

In general

The posture is a variation of vajrasana (p. 97) and may be done with this position as the starting point, either

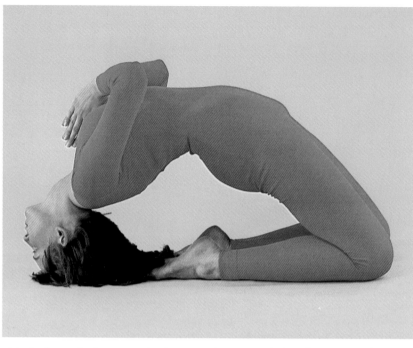

with the buttocks between the feet or sitting on the soles of the feet. When you go into the posture, you should first bend the loins, then the chest, then contract the shoulder blades and, lastly, bend the neck back. In the complete posture breathing should be slow and concentrated in the chest, thereby avoiding tensions in the abdominal and shoulder muscles.

In a few cases you may feel dizzy after having bent the neck back. This will disappear if you put your head down and relax the neck. When you leave the posture, you should first straighten up the body and relax with the forehead on the floor in front of the

knees, and then loosen up the position of the legs. The joints of the knees and ankles are at risk if you try to move the legs in the posture.

In the case of weaknesses in the cervical vertebrae, or dizziness, variation No. 2 should be performed.

Duration

Begin with a few seconds and gradually increase the time to a maximum of a few minutes. If you want to remain for a longer time in the posture, you may lower the head and back in order to lie down flat and relaxed.

Technique

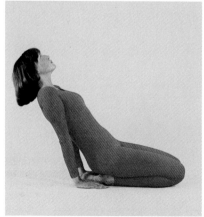

Sit in vajrasana (p. 97) with knees together. Rest the palms of the hands on the floor beside the feet. Arch back slightly from waist to chest.

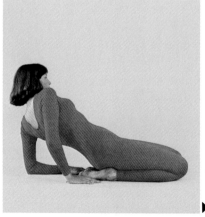

Inhale, relax the right side and rest the right elbow on the floor, then the left elbow. Lift the breast-bone, arching further, bring the shoulder blades together and bend the neck backward.

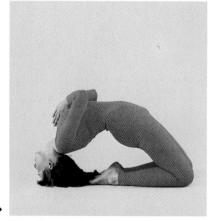

Place the top of the head on the floor and exhale. Lift buttocks and join the palms at the chest. Lower arms and buttocks. Rest on forearms, inhale and lift the head. Come straight up by stretching the arms.

Technique for advanced yoga students

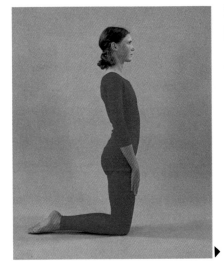 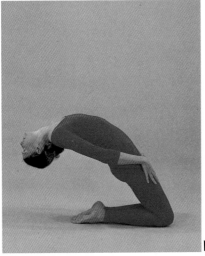 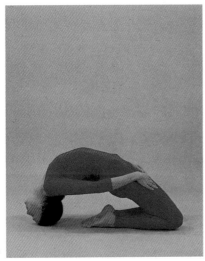

Kneel upright with the palms against the front side of the thighs. Contract buttocks and hamstring muscles, pushing the hips slightly forward.

Inhale and arch the back from the waist upward, raising the breast-bone high. Bring the shoulder blades together, and elongate the neck as you bend the head backward.

Using the muscles of the thighs, continue the movement till the top of the head rests on the floor. Come up by pulling the body upright, or as under technique.

Variations

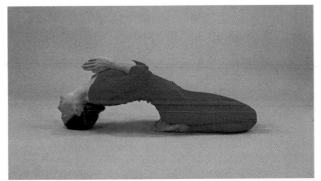 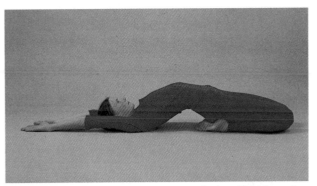

1. Supta vajrasana can be performed resting on the heels until the flexibility of the back and the strength of the thighs have been developed sufficiently for the pose as shown under technqiue.

2. Sit in vajrasana (p. 97), buttocks between the feet. Hold the arches of the feet, lean back carefully and rest on the elbows, lowering the back and neck to the floor. Extend the arms along the head and relax.

Preliminary exercises

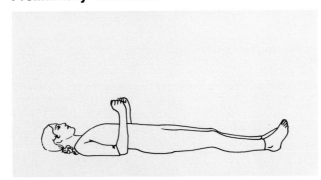 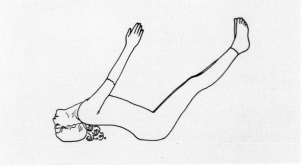

1. Lie on the back with the elbows close to the ribs, feet and forearms vertical, fists clenched . Press the elbows on the floor, lifting the head and back. Stretch the spine, curving back from the waist upward. Contract the shoulder blades lifting the breast-bone, and lower the top of the head on the floor. Breathe quietly. Bend the chin towards the chest and lower the back, vertebra by vertebra.

2. Lie on the back with the arms extended alongside, knees bent and the soles of the feet on the floor. Rest on the elbows, lift the head and back, and arch from waist to neck till the top of the head reaches the floor. If you rest securely on the head, you may extend legs and arms 45°. Place elbows and feet on the floor, lift the head and uncoil the back.

Janu sirshasana

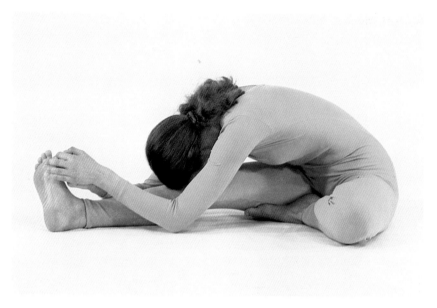

Name

Janu means knee and *sirsha* means head. In this posture the head is resting on the knee of the stretched leg.

Effect

Janu sirshasana may be considered a mild variation of paschin...tanasana (p. 70), and can be done if the latter is too difficult. The posture stretches the muscles of the back and sides in turn. It strengthens and makes supple the back, loins and hips. It prevents lumbago, pains in the loins, and sciatica, and counteracts the formation of abdominal fat. Janu sirshasana gives a strengthening massage to the abdominal organs, but unlike paschimottanasana, the pressure is limited to that side of the body where the leg is extended, while the opposite side is stretched strongly. This alternating pressure-and-stretch effect stimulates circulation of blood in the abdomen, facilitating digestion. In variation No. 2 the spinal column is both stretched and rotated, which stimulates the blood circulation and strengthens the spinal nerves. This posture also stretches the muscles between the ribs and thereby facilitates respiration.

In general

In this position, as in paschimottanasana, you should bend from the hip joint, trying to keep the back straight in order to lessen the strain on the lumbar vertebrae. In the initial phase you draw the abdomen in and up slightly, as in uddiyana (p. 121), but in the complete posture you relax the abdominal muscles so that the stimulating effect on the blood circulation is not inhibited. In this posture, you get the best result if you avoid bending the stretched leg, and if the knee of the other leg remains on the floor. Make sure that both buttocks remain on the floor during the whole exercise, as there may be a tendency to lift the side where the leg is bent. If you want to breathe in the posture, you must be careful to relax the body, otherwise you can easily become short of breath and breathing will be forced. When you come out of the posture, begin by straightening up the hip joint and rolling up the back, vertebra by vertebra. Lastly lift up the head, straighten the body and face forward.

Duration

Begin with a few seconds in the posture, or for so long as it is comfortable to keep the lungs emptied. Gradually you can repeat the exercise a couple of times to each side. If you breathe in the posture, the maximum duration should be a couple of minutes to each side.

Technique

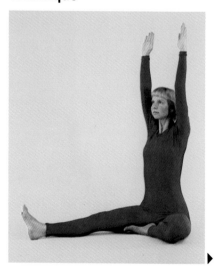

Sit straight with legs extended. Bend the left leg and place the sole of the foot along the right thigh, close to the groin. Move the right leg a little to the side, toes pointing up, and raise the arms above the head.

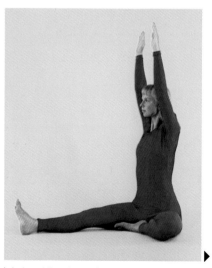

Inhale while elongating and concaving the spine. Face the right leg, and exhale, pulling the abdomen in and bending the pelvis and trunk forward. Keep the spine stretched.

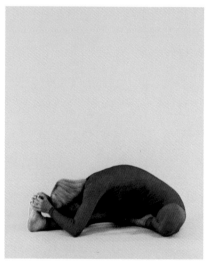

Grasp the toes and lower the trunk and head toward the straight leg. Try to relax, allowing the elbows to sink toward the floor. Slowly unbend and inhale. Repeat to the left.

Variations

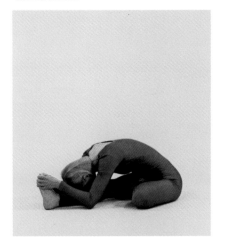

1. Place the left instep in the right groin as in padmasana (p. 112) and perform janu sirshasana as described under technique. Repeat on opposite side.

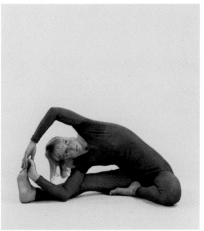

2. With legs as in janu sirshasana, grasp the right foot with the right hand. Inhale, stretching the spine. Exhale bending to the right, elbow toward the floor. Raise the left arm above the head and grasp the right foot. Keep a forward rotation of the trunk.

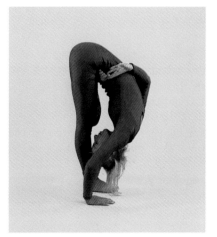

3. Stand up straight and place the left foot in the right groin, bring the left arm round the back and grasp the left foot. Exhale pulling the abdomen in, and bend forward, placing the right palm beside the right foot. Bring the forehead toward the shin.

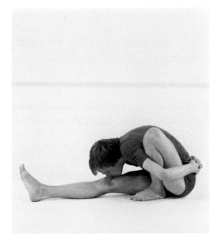

4. Place the left foot on the floor close to the thigh. Bend the left arm round the bent leg and grasp the right hand behind the back. Inhale, stretching the back. Exhale, lowering trunk and head toward the straight leg.

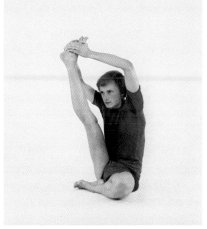

5. Sit with the left heel on the floor close to the groin, the right leg stretched out. Grasp the right foot with both hands. Inhale, straighten the back, exhale, pulling the stretched leg toward trunk and head.

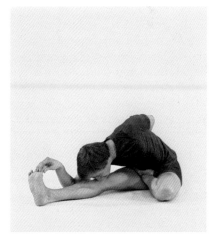

6. Sit with the left foot in the right groin. Move the left arm round the back and grasp the left foot's toes. Grasp the right foot with the right hand, inhale extending the back. Exhale, and bend forward over the right leg.

Preliminary exercises

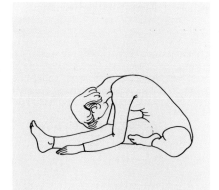

1. With the legs as in janu sirshasana, place the hands on the floor on either side of the extended leg and bend forward in a relaxed way, till the forearms rest on the floor. Relax in the hip joint at each exhalation.

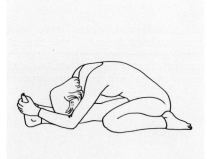

2. Bend the left knee and place the foot by the left hip. Perform janu sirshasana, being careful not to lift the left buttock. Repeat on opposite side. This may be performed in case of weakness in the hip joint or groin.

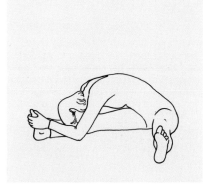

3. In case of weak or stiff knees, you may keep both legs extended wide apart, toes pointing up. If it is not possible to reach the toes with a straight back, you may hold the ankles, calves or knees. Bend over the right leg first, then over the left leg.

Chakrasana

Name

Chakra means wheel. In this asana the body takes the form of a wheel.

Effect

Chakrasana is a posture that keeps the spine supple, strong and healthy. It counteracts a rounded back, gives a more relaxed and correct posture, and alleviates or removes pains in the loins and shoulders. Owing to the weight of the head, a certain lessening of the pressure on the cervical vertebrae is achieved, a pressure which may be inhibiting in the case of muscle tensions. The posture exerts a powerful stretch on the muscles of the front side of the body, especially those of the thighs and abdomen. The abdominal stretch works as a tonic for the internal organs, counteracting tension around the midriff, a sluggish stomach and obesity. If you breathe in this posture, the respiratory muscles are beneficially stretched, just as the heart is massaged, stimulating blood circulation. The posture alleviates headaches, symptoms of weariness and facial tension. It is a stimulating exercise for those who do strenuous intellectual work. In variation No. 3 the diaphragm and the front side of the chest are stretched even more. This exercises the respiratory muscles and helps breathing to become easier and deeper.

In general

Chakrasana presupposes a supple back, strong wrists and a great deal of strength in the arms and legs. To

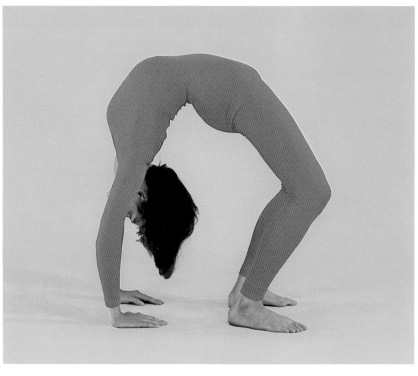

strengthen the wrists you may use the preliminary exercises for mayurasana (p. 73). The posture has the advantage that it may be performed gradually, raising the body increasingly as the back becomes more supple. In the beginning you will feel the stretch in the front thigh muscles, and most experience some soreness, which soon disappears. When you have reached the phase where the arms are stretched, you can increase the effect by tightening the muscles of the buttocks, and stretching the thighs and abdomen upwards. In order to reach the perfect chakrasana you let the hands "walk" towards the feet, then grasp the ankles so that the body forms a full circle.

Care with the posture should be taken in the event of high blood pressure, a weak heart or signs of wear in the spinal column.

Duration

In the beginning it is advisable to remain only a few seconds in the pose and then gradually to prolong the time. You can remain in chakrasana as long as it is comfortable to hold the breath, or you can breathe normally and remain in the position between half a minute and 1 minute.

Technique

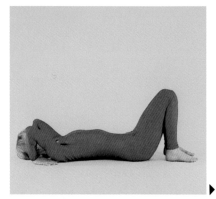

Lie on the back, with feet close to the buttocks, parallel to each other and apart at hip width. Place the palms on the floor under the shoulders, fingers pointing toward the feet.

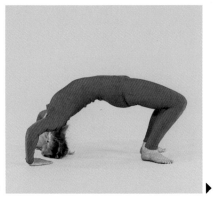

Inhale, tighten the thighs and buttocks, and lift hips and breast-bone high. Push with the palms of the hands and lift the head. Rest the top of the head on the floor, exhaling.

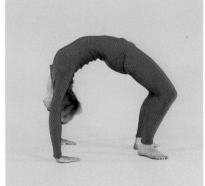

Inhale and stretch the arms. Exhale, arching the body as high as possible. Breathe quietly in the pose. Lift the chin towards the chest, carefully lowering the neck and back. Relax with knees folded on the chest.

Variations

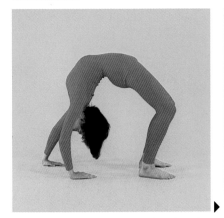

1. Walk the hands closer to the feet, keeping the elevation of the body.

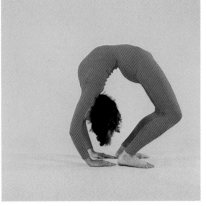

This forms the complete chakrasana, in which the fingers touch the heels, so that the body forms a wheel.

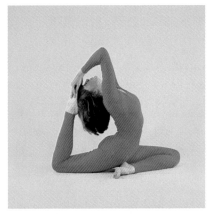

2. Sit with the left leg bent, with the heel touching the right groin. Take the right leg backward, bending the lower leg to vertical. Rest the palms on the floor and inhale. Bend back, exhale and move the left arm over the head to grasp the foot. Catch hold with the right hand too and bring the head to the foot.

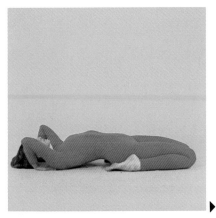

3. Lie on the back, buttocks in between the feet: see supta vajrasana var. No. 2 (p. 75). Place the palms on the floor, fingers under the shoulders.

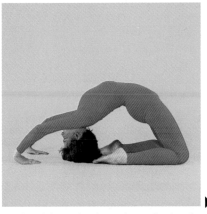

Inhale, tighten the buttocks and raise the hips as you stretch the arms, extending the breast-bone, thereby arching the back. Initially you may rest the top of the head on the floor, then advanced students continue with the next phase.

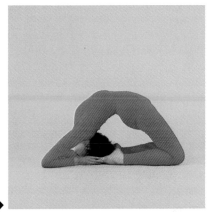

Move hands to feet, rest forearms on the floor. Exhale and lift higher, bringing the top of the head to the feet. Breathe quietly. Bring the palms back onto the floor, bend chin to chest, lowering buttocks and back. Come up and sit as in supta vajrasana (p. 74).

Preliminary exercises

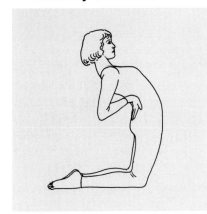

1. Kneel upright. Support the small of the back with the palms. Tighten the muscles of the thighs and buttocks, pushing thighs and hips forward. Curve backward from the lumbar region upward, extend breast-bone and bring shoulder blades together.

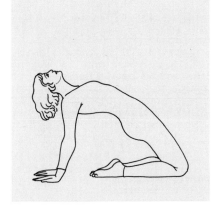

2. Sit in vajrasana, palms on floor behind feet. Inhale, contract buttocks and thighs, raising the hips high. Flex from the lumbar vertebrae upward, bring the shoulder blades together and bend the head back. Bend chin to the chest and lower buttocks.

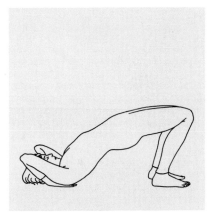

3. Starting position as in chakrasana. Inhale, tighten the thighs and buttocks, lifting the buttocks and back off the floor. Exhale, raising hips and breast-bone higher. Inhale and lower the spine vertebra by vertebra. Relax in pavanamuktasana var. No. 1 (p. 82).

Kandharasana

Name

Kandhar means shoulder. In kandharasana a large part of the body rests on the shoulders.

Effect

Kandharasana strengthens the spinal column and makes it supple, counteracting a rounded back and sagging shoulders. It strengthens the muscles of the legs, back and buttocks, makes the hip joints supple and removes tension in the neck and the front of the body. The respiratory muscles receive a relaxing stretch, and the heart and blood circulation are stimulated. Kandharasana facilitates the return of venous blood from the abdomen, counteracting venous stasis in the abdominal organs and also haemorrhoids. The posture also increases the circulation of blood to the head and neck, leading to a refreshing effect.

In general

If it is difficult for you to reach the ankles with the hands, you can initially draw the bent legs close to the body, grasp the ankles and then put the feet on the floor. Take care that the neck remains straight.

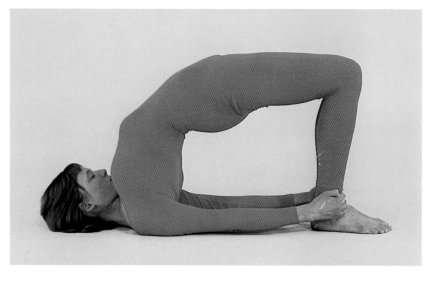

In order to achieve the greatest benefit, try to lift the body by means of the thigh and buttock muscles, without using the muscles of the back until the end. While standing in the posture, the neck muscles must be relaxed, so that the stretching effect can work, and lessen the pressure between the vertebrae. If you breathe while in the pose, you can try to press the abdomen further upwards in the interval between inhalation and exhalation. The exercise is concluded by letting go of the ankles, inhaling and lowering the back, vertebra by vertebra. When the buttocks are down, the legs are stretched, so in order to relax the calf muscles, you can bend the instep towards the knees. In the case of a hollow back, the loins may be relaxed by bending the knees towards the chest.

Duration

Begin with a couple of seconds in the posture and repeat it twice. Gradually increase the time to 2 minutes.

Technique

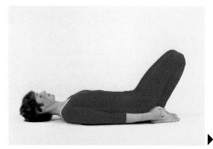

Lie on the back with legs bent, feet together close to the buttocks. Grasp the ankles and tuck in the chin, keeping the neck straight.

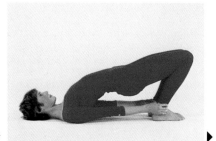

Inhale, tighten the thigh muscles and lift buttocks and spine from the floor, one vertebra at a time.

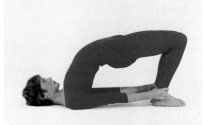

Exhale, arching as high as possible. Raise the breast-bone, and tighten the buttocks, lifting higher with each breath. Inhale and roll down the spine vertebra by vertebra.

Preliminary exercises

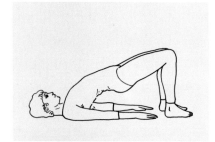

1. Perform the pose with the feet a hip width apart, slightly behind the buttocks, and the arms on the floor along the sides of the body.

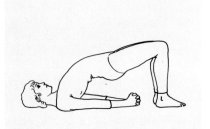

2. Commence as in No. 1, with legs together or apart. Interlock the fingers and pull the hands and shoulders toward the feet, arching the body higher.

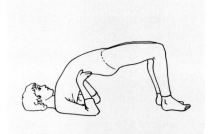

3. Enter the pose as described. Support the lower back with the hands, keeping elbows close and shoulder blades together. Lower the arms and slowly uncoil the back.

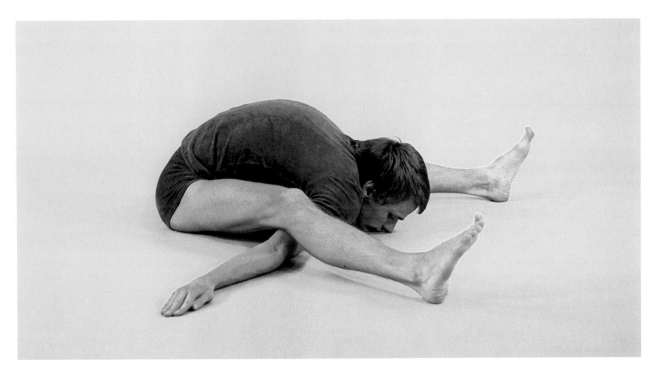

Name

Kurmasana means the tortoise posture.

Effect

Kurmasana is a good stretching exercise that keeps the whole of the spinal column healthy and supple. By placing the arms under the legs the stretch between the vertebrae is increased, improving metabolism in the vertebral discs and increasing blood circulation in the back. The posture gives suppleness in the hip and pelvic area, strengthens the abdominal muscles and stimulates the organs of the abdomen. Kurmasana stretches and relaxes the upper back muscles, the buttock muscles, and the inner thigh muscles. It has a good effect on the nervous system, leading to an increase in physical energy and elimination of fatigue and pain in the loins. Kurmasana counteracts restlessness, mental strain and nervousness, and assists in turning the mind to inner contemplation.

In general

Begin with the first phase of the technique. Avoid bending too much in the loins, but try to keep the spine straight and bend forward from the hips. Relax the hip joints and let go with every exhalation. Keep the head up and stretch the chin forward, so that you keep the spinal column as straight as possible. It is important not to use force to press the body into this posture as this may strain the spinal column and lead to painful overstretching of the muscles.

Duration

Remain in the posture so long as it is comfortable to hold the breath after exhaling, or breathe normally a couple of times. Gradually increase the time up to two minutes, breathing calmly.

Technique

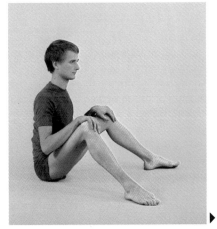

Sit with legs bent and spread apart, hands on knees. Inhale stretching the spine, raise the breast-bone and push back the shoulders.

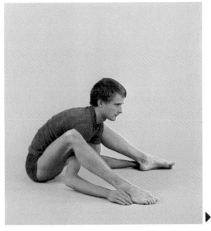

Exhale, pull in the abdomen and bend pelvis and trunk forward. Place the elbows on the floor under the knees and slide the arms out sideways under the legs.

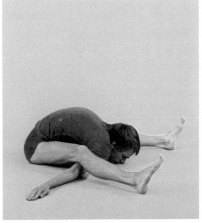

Slowly stretch out the legs, and lower the body to the floor, extending chin and breast-bone. Relax. Bring the feet back, bending at the knees, pull back the arms and straighten up.

Pavanamuktasana

Name

Pavana means wind. *Mukta* means free.

Effect

Pavanamuktasana stimulates the digestive organs, and is particularly suitable in removing air from the intestines. The posture has a special effect on these organs and alleviates constipation. Pavanamuktasana stretches the muscles in the loins, buttocks and thighs. It makes the hip and knee joints supple, counteracts pain and tension in the loins, and effectively prevents downward curvature of the spine. The horizontal variations are also effective relaxation exercises for an overstrained and tired back.

In general

In the beginning it is difficult for most people to get the thighs close to the body. If you relax in the posture and perform it regularly, the suppleness will soon come. Take care that the neck remains straight and shoulders and loins are relaxed. Owing to the pressure on the lower part of the intestinal canal, the right leg is bent first and then the left. Ensure that the knee does not slip to one side when you do the exercise with one leg at a time. When both legs are bent towards the chest, the knees are kept together and the hips remain on the floor, so that the back remains straight. In the static posture you should breathe as deeply as possible, in order to strengthen the effect on the digestive organs. However, to avoid tension do not overdo it. The

Technique

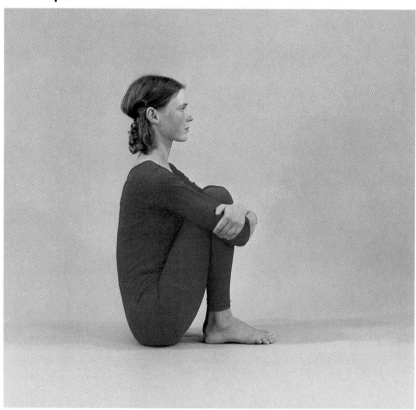

Sit up straight. Bring the knees up to the chest, keeping the legs together and the feet on the floor. Fold the arms around the knees, grasping the opposite elbow. Straighten up the back, bringing trunk and thighs close together. Remain for a while in the pose, as relaxed as possible, and concentrate on breathing slowly and deeply.

horizontal variation may also be done as a dynamic exercise: inhale and bend the right knee towards the chest. Fold the hands around the knee and press the thigh against the body. Exhale and lift the forehead to the knee. Then lower the head and inhale, stretch the leg out and exhale. Repeat with the left leg, and lastly with both legs. This is a beneficial warming-up exercise to do prior to commencing the static yoga postures, provided that the movements are carried out smoothly.

Duration

Giving equal time to every phase, pavanamuktasana may be done so long as there is no discomfort. The dynamic variation may be repeated 3-5 times.

Variations

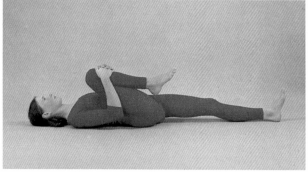

1. Lie on the back with the legs a hip-width apart. Bend the right leg to the right chest, interlock the fingers round the knee and relax. Repeat with the left leg bent, then with both legs.

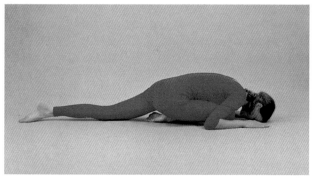

2. Rest on knees and hands. Extend the left leg backward and lower the buttocks on the right heel, so the body is resting on the right thigh, the knee toward the right chest. Relax with the forehead on the floor. Repeat with the left leg bent, and with both legs.

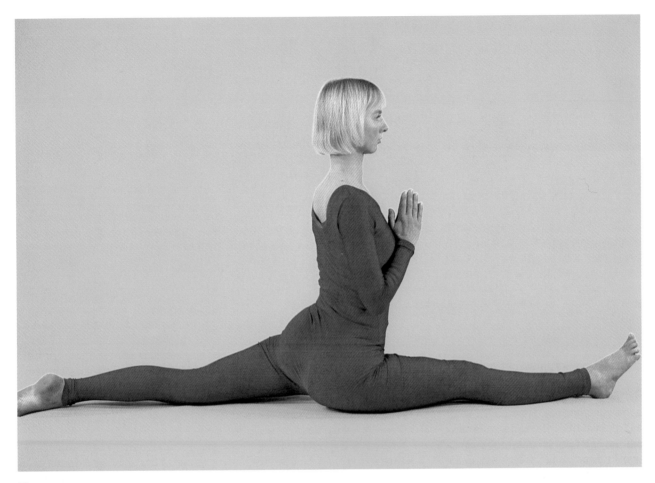

Name

Hanuman is a mythological hero who crossed the straits between India and Sri Lanka in one single leap.

Effect

Hanumanasana strengthens and makes supple the hips and pelvic area and removes abdominal tension. The posture stretches the muscles in the legs, buttocks and hips, stimulates blood circulation in the legs and abdo-men and helps to keep these parts healthy. If the arms are stretched over the head, a powerful stretching of the body is achieved, and this may remove or alleviate back pains.

In general

It is important to prepare for hanu-manasana very carefully to avoid over-stretching. This is done by practising the first two phases of the technique.

Hold back by putting the weight on the arms and relax the hips, pelvic floor and legs. The suppleness cannot be forced, but it will come gradually when you relax sufficiently. Go back to the starting posture by resting on the hands and the back knee, and by drawing in the front foot towards the hands.

Duration

As long as it is comfortable.

Technique

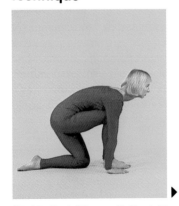

Rest on the left knee with the right foot on the floor so the shin is vertical. Place both hands on either side of the right foot.

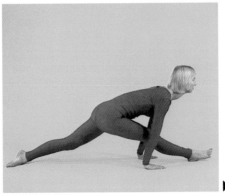

Inhale, extend the right leg forward and the left leg backward. Exhale, sliding the feet over the floor. Keep the weight of the body on the hands while carefully lowering the legs.

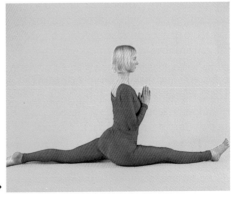

When both legs are stretched and resting on the floor, straighten the back and bring the palms together in front of the chest, or overhead. Repeat on the other side.

Gomukhasana

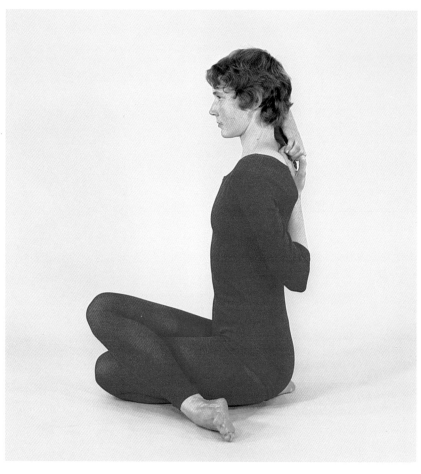

Name

Gomukh is the name of a classical Indian musical instrument, the form of which resembles a cow.

Effect

Gomukhasana makes the shoulder joints supple, stretches the muscles of the upper arms and back, and offsets tension and rheumatic pains in the shoulders, arms and back. The posture counteracts stoop and gives a graceful pose. The chest is expanded by stretching the large chest muscle and the rib muscles. This increases the lung capacity, counteracts ailments of the air passages and makes breathing free and easy. Furthermore, gomukhasana relaxes the abdominal muscles and is well known as a help in alleviating haemorrhoids, enteritis and constipation. Stretching the buttocks and thighs is particularly effective in relieving sciatica and rheumatism in the legs. The forward-bend variation may alleviate headaches and sinusitis, and will open up the nasal passages if the nostrils are blocked owing to colds. This posture is also recommended in cases of insomnia, owing to its considerable relaxing effect.

In general

If you suffer from varicose veins or bad knees, the posture may be done standing or kneeling. In order not to overstrain the joints, avoid sudden movements in the initial or exit phases. Be particularly careful if you have loose joint ligaments or osteoarthritis in the hips or shoulders. In the complete posture, neck and back should be straight, the arms free of the head and the knees right over each other. If the shoulders and arms are sore after the posture, you can conclude with shoulder exercises Nos. 8 and 9 (p. 32).

Duration

Begin by sitting for a few seconds in the posture and gradually increase the time to two minutes on each side.

Technique

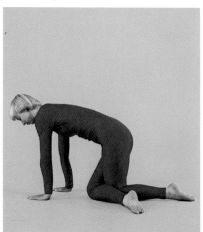

Rest on hands and knees. Bring the right leg across the left one and lower the buttocks so that the left heel is against the anus. Keep the right foot close to the left hip and the knees just over each other.

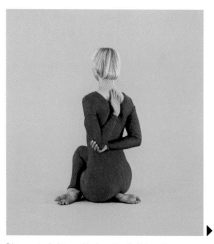

Sit up straight and bring the left hand up your back, palm outward. Pull the left elbow towards the centre of the back, with the hand reaching as high as possible.

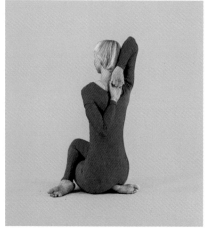

Raise the right arm overhead. Bend the elbow and grasp the left hand. Try to keep the right arm behind the head. Sit with a straight back, breathing deeply and regularly. Repeat on opposite side.

Variations

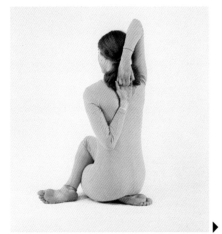 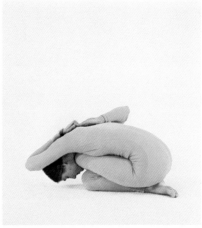 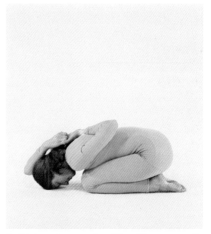

1. Sit erect in gomukhasana. Inhale while concaving the back.

Exhale, tuck in the stomach and bend forward from the hips until the chin reaches outside the knees. Relax, lowering the head toward the floor. Repeat on the opposite side.

2. Sit in vajrasana (p. 97), with arms as in gomukhasana. Inhale, stretching the spine. Exhale bending forward, and place the forehead on the floor. Relax, avoiding lifting the buttocks.

Preliminary exercises

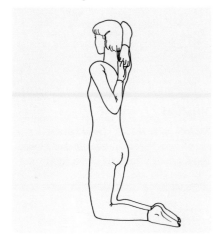 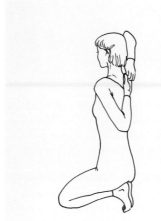 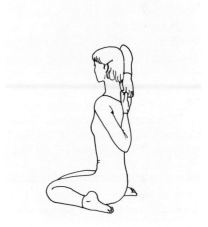

1. If the hips are weak or stiff, the arm position may be performed kneeling.

2. Perform the arm pose sitting in vajrasana. Curl the toes under as shown if the calves tend to cramp.

3. Perform the pose with the buttocks on the floor in between the feet. The toes may point straight backward or out to either side.

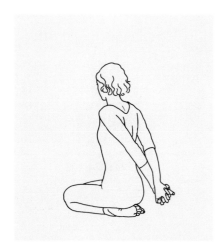 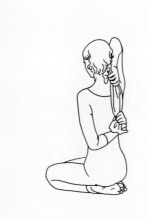 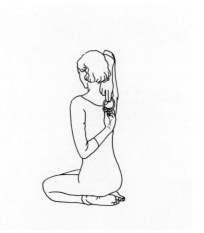

4. Sit straight, wrists crossed behind the back and fingers interlocked. Inhale, pull the arms down and backward, bringing the shoulder blades together. Relax and exhale.

5. While practising the arm position, hold a scarf or something similar, gradually diminishing the distance between the hands.

6. Or the pose may be carried out holding a ring, if the hands do not meet. The arm positions shown may be practised in any leg position, keeping a straight back.

Chatuskonasana

Name

Chatuskonasana means four-cornered posture.

Effect

This asana makes the hip joints supple, stretches the muscles of the buttocks and the hollows of the knees, and massages the internal organs. The combined pressure-and-stretch effect stimulates blood circulation and the nervous system, so that you feel refreshed and really recharged with physical as well as mental energy.

In general

It may be beneficial to prepare for chatuskonasana by doing the preliminary exercises for padmasana (p. 113) and akarna dhanurasana (p. 87). It is wise to spend sufficient time in preparation, not trying to complete the posture until you have gained the necessary suppleness. If you proceed too quickly, overstretching of the buttocks and backs of the knees may follow. In the beginning, chatuskonasana may cause a rapid quickening of the pulse, an increase in body heat and irregular breathing. After a little practice, you learn to control the

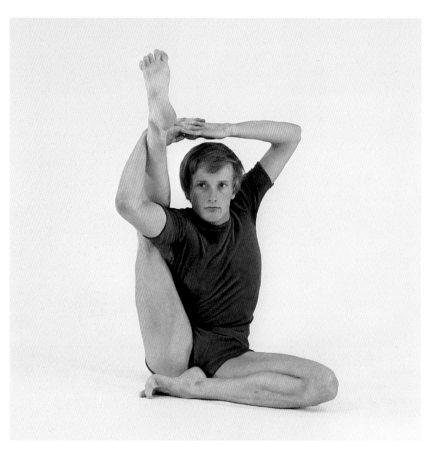

liberated energy (prana) and to enjoy the resulting fitness.

Duration

At first remain in the position for a couple of seconds, then, if you feel good, gradually extend the time.

Technique

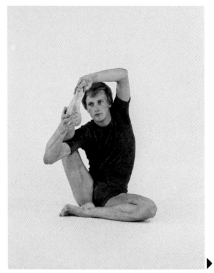

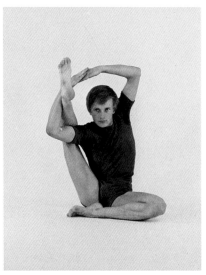

Sit with the left leg bent, heel close to the groin. Lift the right leg and place the hollow of the knee to the right elbow joint.

Move the leg upwards until it rests on the shoulder. Bring both hands together above the head and straighten up the back. Repeat on the other side.

Variation

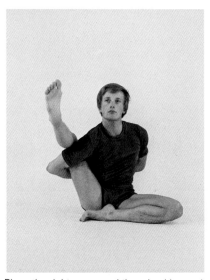

Place the right arm round the raised leg and clasp the left hand behind the back. Keep the back straight. Repeat on the other side.

Name

Dhanurasana means bow position. *Akarna* means ear. In this exercise the foot is drawn up towards the ear like the arrow on a bowstring.

Effect

This is an effective exercise to make the hips and legs supple, and at the same time to strengthen the muscles of the arms, shoulders and back. Akarna dhanurasana is a remedy for sciatica-type pains, where these are due to tight muscles; it also relaxes the muscles of the buttocks and thighs. The alternate contraction and stretching of the muscles in the shoulders and back counteracts and prevents symptoms of tension which are very frequent in these areas. The pressure of the thighs on the abdomen stimulates the internal organs and digestion, and acts as a corrective for abdominal fat. The posture counteracts restlessness and stress, giving calmness and vitality to body and mind.

In general

Remember that it is the foot that is going up to the ear, and not vice versa. It is a common error to bend forwards in order to get the foot up to the ear. The posture is most effective when you keep the back, neck and head straight.

Breathing should be deep and calm. Avoid drawing the leg so high that

Technique

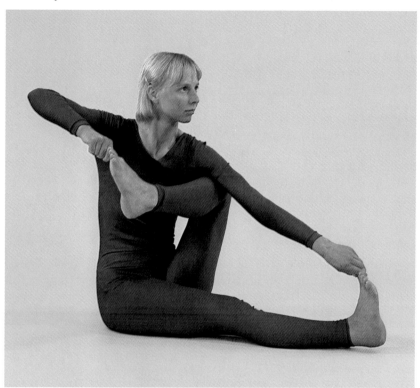

Sit erect, legs stretched out. Place the left foot on the right thigh, and grasp the foot with the right hand. Keep the right knee straight, bend the ankle and grasp the right big toe with the left hand. Using the right hand, lift the left leg until the knee reaches the left armpit. Inhale, stretch the spine and pull the left foot towards the right ear, moving the right elbow backwards. Repeat to the opposite side.

you become short of breath owing to strain, or that you feel pain in the joints. Knee and hip joints can be made supple by the preliminary exercises shown here, and also through the preliminary exercises for padmasana (p. 113). Always begin by lifting the right leg first and then repeat with the left.

Duration

Take 2 to 6 calm breaths in the posture and then repeat on the opposite side.

Variations

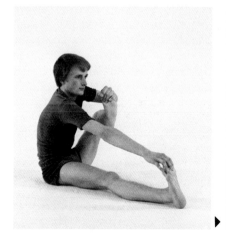

Grasp the left foot with the left hand, and the right foot with the right hand. Bend the left leg backward and pull the foot toward the left ear.

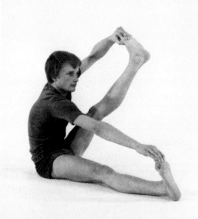

Try to straighten up the back. Extend the raised leg toward the ceiling. Repeat with the right leg.

Preliminary exercises

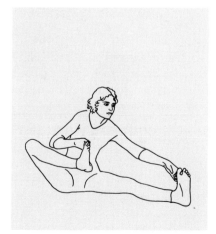

Sit with the legs extended a hip width apart. Stretch the spine, bend forward and grasp the feet with both hands. Bend the right leg and, using the right hand, pull the knee backward and outward. Repeat to the left.

Samkatasana

Name

The word *samkat* means tight, closed, difficult and dangerous. In samkatasana the legs are closed tightly around the pelvis.

Effect

This posture makes the joints of the hips and knees supple and strong. It stretches the thighs and buttocks forcefully, which effectively alleviates sciatic pains. The small of the back is almost automatically straightened up, thus ensuring good back posture, which may help to alleviate pain and to correct curvature of the spine and a faulty carriage. Samkatasana may be considered a kind of mudra or seal (p. 119), which, in connection with mula bandha (p. 120), gives a tonic to the lower pelvis and the abdominal organs, at the same time regulating nervousness in this area. The posture therefore has the effect of maintaining the pelvic organs in good condition, and may help to control sexual energy.

In the dynamic variations all the muscles of the back are exercised and strenghtened, the shoulders are relaxed and the internal organs beneficially massaged.

In general

Be careful with this posture. In particular, avoid sudden jerky move-

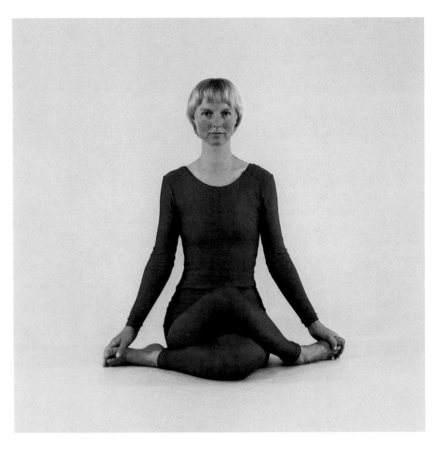

ments to force the legs into position, as this may result in overstrain and damage to the joints of the knees and hips. If painful, the posture should be relaxed. Take care not to lift the hip on the side where the leg is uppermost, and keep the spine quite straight. In the perfect pose the knees are just on top of each other and the heels are close to the body.

Duration

So long as it is comfortable and for the same time with each leg uppermost.

Technique I

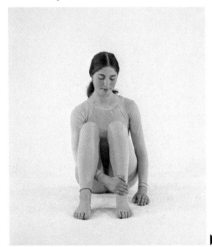

Sit with legs bent. Bring the right hand underneath the right leg and catch hold of the left ankle.

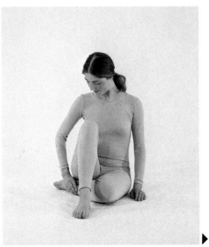

Pull the left leg under the right leg, and place the left heel close to the right hip.

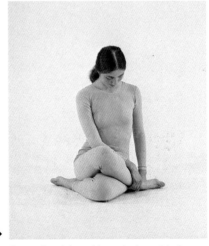

Grasp the right ankle and place this leg so the heel is lying close to the left hip and the knees are exactly above each other. Place hands on feet and extend the back.

Technique II

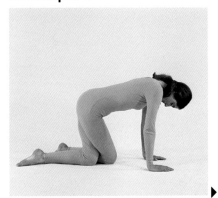 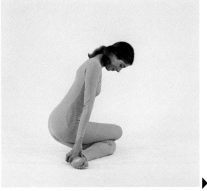 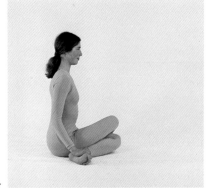

Rest on hands and knees. Cross the right leg in over the left knee.

Grasp both heels and place the buttocks exactly in the middle between the feet. The weight of the body should remain on hands and feet.

Lower the buttocks cautiously, transferring the weight equally to both seat bones. Sit with a straight back. Repeat with the left leg above.

Variations

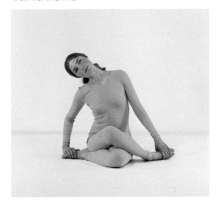 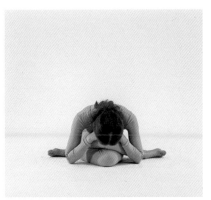 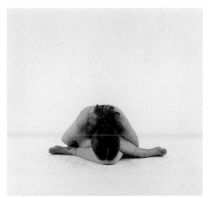

1. Inhale and bend from the waist straight down to the side of the lower foot. Exhale and relax, going deeper into the movement. Come up straight and inhale.

2. Place both hands on the knees. Inhale, extend the back. Exhale, bending forward till the chin reaches outside the knees, and the elbows rest on the floor. Relax.

3. As in the previous variation, with both hands behind the buttocks, chin outside the knees and forehead towards the floor. Relax in the pose. Repeat on opposite side.

Preliminary exercises

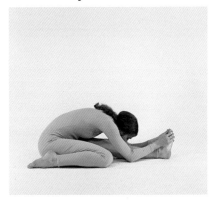 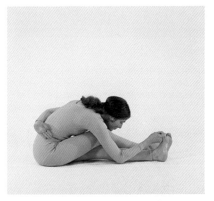 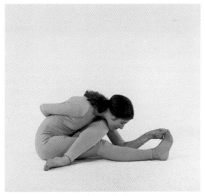

1. Sit with legs stretched in front, a hip width apart. Bend one leg to the side and place the foot by the hip. Inhale, elongate and concave the spine. Exhale, bend forward over the extended leg with back straight, and grasp the foot. Relax, lowering the elbows to the floor.

2. Cross the right leg over the left one, so the knees are above each other. Bring the left arm behind the lower back. Inhale concaving the spine. Exhale and bend forward till the chin is outside the knees and the right hand grasps the left foot. Relax, lowering the elbow toward the floor.

3. Perform this variation in the same way as the preceding one, only with the upper leg bent and the heel close to the thigh of the extended leg. Repeat all these exercises with the opposite leg stretched out.

Mandukasana

Name

Mandukasana means frog posture.

Effect

Mandukasana is a kneeling posture which is often used for meditation and breathing exercises. It facilitates keeping a straight back and may remove from the loins and back the pains which prevent many from sitting in other meditation postures. Further, it makes the ankles, knees and hips supple, stretches the thigh muscles, and, in part, those of the abdomen. The variation with separate knees increases the stretching effect and counteracts abdominal tension. The dynamic series stretches the back and the muscles of the buttocks, and alleviates tension in the shoulders and neck. This series may cure headaches and in some cases will prevent migraine. Be careful in the case of loose joint ligaments in the shoulders.

In general

The posture may be prepared for by doing leg exercise No. 6 (p. 41), and vajrasana (p. 97) or bhadrasana (p. 107). In the dynamic series of exercises it is important to keep the sway in the loin and between the shoulder blades. Initially most people find it difficult to reach the floor. Suppleness will come gradually when you relax and give in with the shoulders.

Duration

As long as it feels comfortable.

Technique

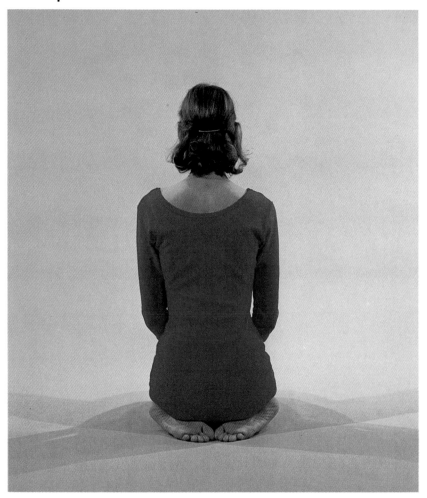

Kneel upright with big toes together and the heels pointing out to either side. Lower the buttocks on the floor between the heels. The knees may be kept together or wide apart. Place hands on thighs, so the elbows are vertically below the shoulders, and extend the breast-bone a little to straighten the spine. Elongate the neck and lower the shoulders. Remain as relaxed as possible with back straight. Breathe slowly and deeply.

Dynamic variation

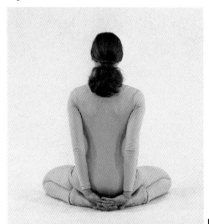

Sit in mandukasana with a straight back and knees wide apart. Interlock the fingers behind the back, palms upturned. Pull the arms downward, bringing the shoulder blades together.

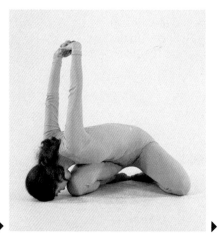

Inhale and turn to the right. Exhale, bending over the right leg and place the forehead on the floor. Raise the arms to vertical. Inhale, lower the arms, lift the head and straighten up. Repeat to the left side.

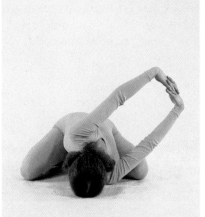

Bend straight forward. Raise both arms and alternately move them to each side, lowering the shoulders toward the floor while keeping the head still. Bring the arms to vertical and lower them. Come up with back straight.

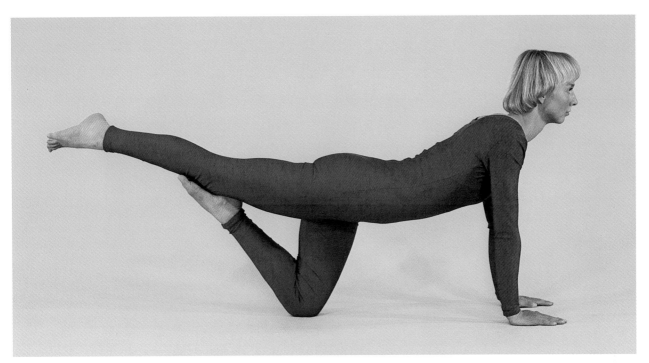

Name

Kutilangasana means snake posture.

Effect

The posture strengthens the muscles of the arms, shoulders, back and buttocks, and it counteracts pain in the loins and back. Phase 2 of the technique makes the loins supple and stretches the thighs and hips, as well as the abdominal muscles. It further stimulates blood circulation, reducing pressure and tension in the lower part of the body. In stretching one arm forward in the final posture, concentration and balance are developed.

In general

Kutilangasana requires a great deal of strength in the wrists; you may use the preliminary training exercises for mayurasana (p. 73). If the wrists become sore, it may help to turn the finger-tips outwards to the sides. If you do not have enough strength in the arms, practise for some time with back exercise No. 4 (p. 37). The posture requires an extra mat to avoid too much pressure on the knees. In the final pose the chest is pushed forward and the shoulders lowered.

Duration

2-6 deep breaths in the complete posture.

Technique

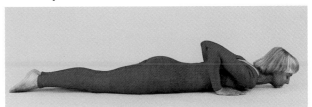

Lie flat on the stomach, palms flat on the floor beside the chest.

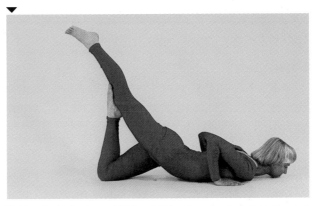

Tighten the buttocks and lift the right leg, keeping it straight. Bend at the left knee, and place the right knee in the arch of the left foot.

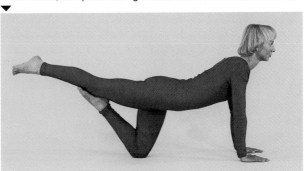

Inhale and push up on both arms, raising the body from the floor, and exhale. Try to stretch the left arm forward. Repeat on the other side.

91

Ustrasana

Name

Ustrasana means camel posture.

Effect

This posture stretches the front of the body from the thighs to the neck, and releases abdominal and respiratory muscle tension. The chest muscles are stretched powerfully, which counteracts sagging shoulders. The exercise strengthens the thigh muscles, buttocks and back, making the spinal column supple and alleviating back pain and particularly tension between the shoulder blades. In the relaxing phase the whole area feels pleasantly warm, as a result of improved blood circulation and metabolism of the muscles and vertebral discs. If the exercise is done regularly, static pressure on the pelvis may decrease, menstrual pains be alleviated and digestion improved.

In general

Ustrasana may be used as a counterpart to *sarvangasana* (p. 54). It is one of the backward positions within the scope of most people. Until the back is supple, you may keep the knees apart with the ankles and toes bent forward. The same position of the feet may be used if you are prone to cramp in the calf muscles. Initially, when the buttocks are lifted, the thigh muscles are used as much as possible, followed by the muscles of the back and buttocks. In the final pose the thighs are vertical and the abdomen is pushed forward by tightening the buttocks and pelvic floor. Draw the shoulder blades together, before lowering the neck backwards, thereby avoiding pressure to the neck. If dizziness is experienced, try to exhale while the head is bent backwards. If this does not help, and if there is any weakness in the cervical vertebrae, keep the head lifted up in the posture. After practising for some time the palms may rest on the soles of the feet, as shown in the main illustration.

Deep calm breathing in the posture effectively massages the abdominal organs. Afterwards, relax the shoulders and loins by resting with the buttocks on the heels, and the forehead on the floor in front of the knees. Be careful with ustrasana if you suffer from hernia or any weakness of the spinal column.

Duration

Begin the posture with a single calm breath. Gradually increase the time up to 1-2 minutes.

Technique I

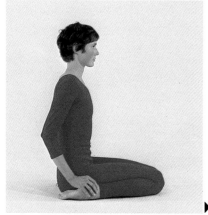

Sit in vajrasana (p. 97), buttocks on the floor between the feet. Place hands on heels. Inhale. Tighten thighs and buttocks, tipping the pelvis backward.

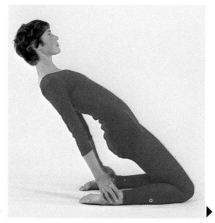

Raise the thighs and buttocks. Move the hips forward, until the thighs are perpendicular, while arching the spine backward from waist to chest. Raise the breast-bone high.

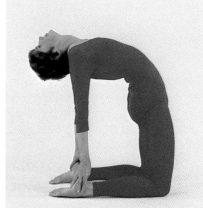

Bring the shoulder blades together and bend back the neck when exhaling. Breathe quietly, lifting upwards with each breath. Inhale, raise the head and lower the buttocks. Exhale and relax with forehead on the floor in front of the knees.

Technique II

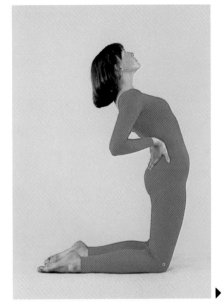 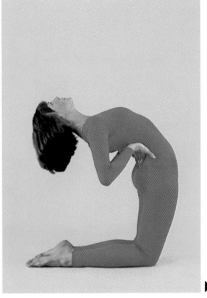 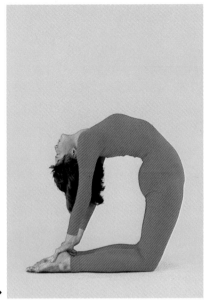

Kneel upright, the knees together and toes pointing back. Support the small of the back with the palms, tighten the buttocks and push the thighs and hips forward.

Inhale and arch the spine, vertebra by vertebra from waist to chest. Bring the shoulder blades together, raising the breast-bone, and arch further backward.

Grasp the heels, move the hips forward and bend the neck backward. Exhale and arch the body higher with each breath. Raise the head and stretch upright. Sit on both heels and relax with forehead on the floor.

Preliminary exercises

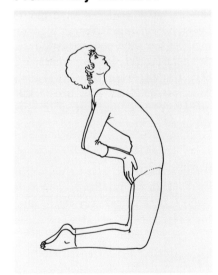 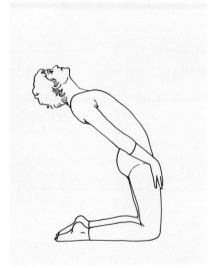 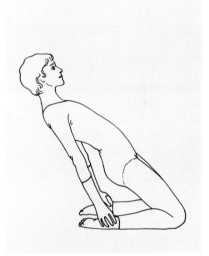

1. Kneel upright with legs a hip-width apart and the palms on the buttocks. Tighten thighs and buttocks, pushing the hips forward. Bend back from waist to chest raising the breast-bone high. Bring the shoulder blades together and bend the neck backwards. Raise the head and straighten up. Relax, resting on both heels, forehead on the floor.

2. Place the palms on top of the thighs. Tense both thighs and buttocks, pushing hips forward, and arch back from waist to chest. Raise the breast-bone and lean back as far as possible. Incline the chin towards the chest and straighten up.

3. Perform ustrasana with legs a hip-width apart. If the calves tend to cramp or if there is any difficulty in reaching the heels with the hands, bend the ankles and turn the toes forwards.

Setuasana

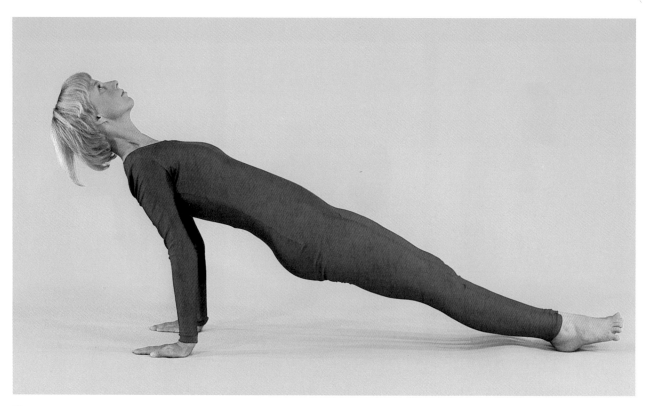

Name

Setuasana means bridge posture.

Effect

Setuasana strengthens the muscles in the legs, buttocks, back and arms; also the wrists, ankles and shoulder joints, and gives a good poise. The posture, especially the variation, which is a little more difficult, stretches the muscles on the front of the body, removes tension in the respiratory muscles and improves the breathing. Setuasana is an effective supplement to the forward-bending postures, especially if the more vigorous backward-bending ones are too difficult.

In general

In this posture, while the breast-bone is raised, you should keep the shoulders lowered and drawn backwards. Take care that the head does not fall back. Tighten the muscles of the buttocks so that they do not sink down. In the variation, first tighten the buttocks and the pelvic floor, and then press the abdomen upwards while the back is curved from the loins to the thoracic vertebrae. It is important to draw the shoulder blades together before the head is bent backwards, in order to avoid pressure on the neck. If you have a tendency to become dizzy, avoid tilting the head backwards. While coming out of the pose the head is first raised, and the buttocks slowly lowered.

Duration

Remain in the posture for up to a minute, breathing deeply and calmly.

Technique

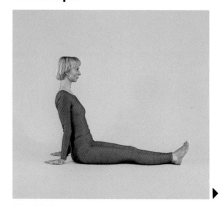

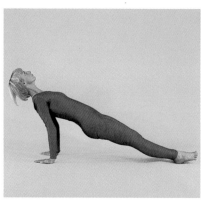

Sit with legs extended and together. Place palms on the floor below the shoulders, finger-tips backwards. Lower the shoulders and raise the breast-bone, straightening the back. Inhale.

Tighten the muscles of buttocks and legs, and raise the body until it forms a straight line from feet to head. The weight is resting on hands and heels. Breathe normally.

Variation

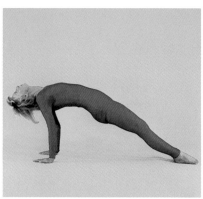

Tighten buttocks and back muscles even more, arching the body upwards. Bring the shoulder blades together and bend the neck back. Keep shoulders low and breast-bone high.

94

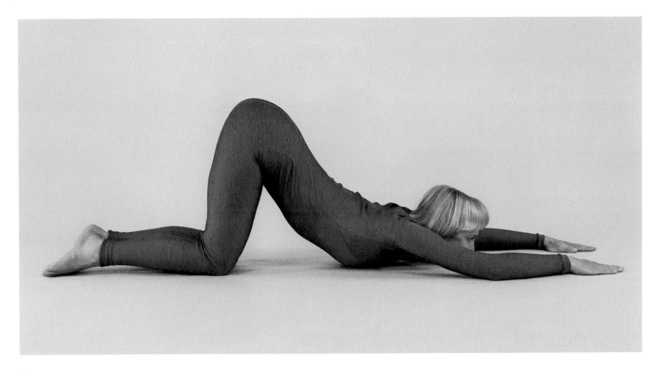

Name

Uttan means stretching, *pristha* means back. The posture is usually called the stretching of the back or "the dog's stretch".

Effect

As the name implies, this is a stretching exercise for the whole of the back, particularly for the spinal column. It is a posture that effectively neutralises pains related to tiredness and tension in the back, neck, shoulders and upper arms, and it is one of the exercises that reaches inflammation between the shoulder blades. Uttan pristhasana makes the back supple, strengthens the muscles of the buttocks and thighs, and stretches the muscles of the abdomen. It stimulates blood supply to the upper part of the body and neck, and reduces abdominal tension and venous stasis. It is a very refreshing posture which may beneficially be done several times a day.

In general

In this posture you must try to relax in the back and between the shoulder blades and "give in„ after each relaxation, so that the breast-bone sinks down on the floor. If any pains arise in the arms and shoulders, it may be helpful to bend the elbows slightly out to the sides. If you feel strain in the back, you should not remain in the position, but slowly slide forward until you are lying flat. If you cannot draw the buttocks back to the initial posture by using the muscles of the buttocks and thighs alone, bend with the arms and push with the hands, after which you can ease back on the heels and rest with the forehead on the floor.

Duration

From half a minute to 2 minutes.

Technique

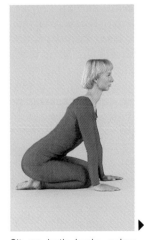

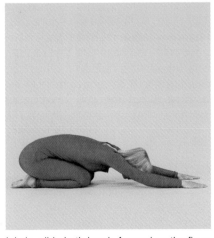

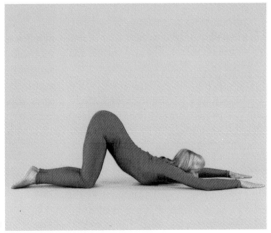

Sit on both heels, palms on the floor alongside the knees. Look forwards, extend the breast-bone, concaving the spine.

Inhale, slide both hands forward on the floor, and stretch as far as possible without lifting the buttocks. Exhale.

Look forward and inhale. Continue sliding forward until both chin and chest rest on the floor. Breathe quietly in the pose and try to relax with each exhalation. Slide further to lie face down, or pull the buttocks back to rest on the heels.

Simhasana

Name

Simhasana means the lion posture.

Effect

Simhasana is really a *bandha* (see p. 119). Owing to contraction of the arms, neck and body in the static position, also the extended tongue, widely open eyes and splayed fingers, the subtle nerve energy, prana (see p. 158), is blocked. However, in the succeeding relaxation phase, this nerve energy is released and flows to the upper part of the body, neck and head. The vitalising effect of simhasana is both physical and mental and may help to alleviate a negative, depressed state of mind.

The posture benefits the whole neck area. It strengthens muscles and tendons, increases blood circulation, regulates the production of saliva and counteracts hoarseness. Simhasana relieves throat pains and is a remedy for inflammation of the throat and tonsils. It may greatly assist people with a dry, nervous cough.

In general

Simhasana requires no special suppleness or training, and may be carried out in any sitting posture. In the main illustration the legs are placed in padmasana (p. 112), with the weight resting on the hands and knees, the buttock muscles tightened and the back and hip joints straightened. This variation makes the hips and loins supple.

As you become accustomed to the posture as described under technique, try a slightly more difficult breathing method. Inhale as described, bend the chin towards the chest while the tongue is extended and the upper part of the body tensed. Hold your breath as long as it feels comfortable, then lift the head and exhale while the body is relaxed.

Duration

Repeat the exercise 3-5 times. In case of a sore throat you may benefit by doing such a series up to 3 times a day.

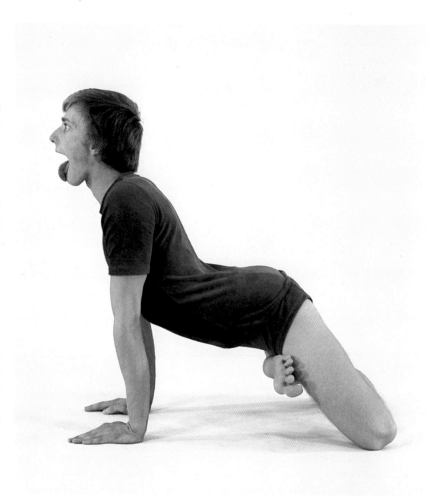

Technique

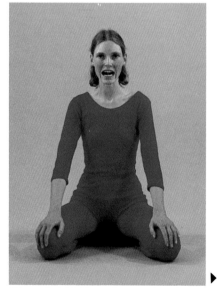

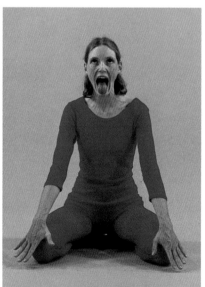

Sit up straight. Open the mouth and place the tip of the tongue behind the upper front teeth. Suck the tongue flat against the palate, until a pull in the ligament under the tongue is noticed and the tendons of the throat protrude. Inhale through the nose.

Exhale vigorously extending the tongue towards the chin as far as possible. At the same time, tighten the neck, upper trunk and arms with fingers extended, open the eyes wide and look up. Relax and inhale quietly through the nose.

Name

Vajra is the name of the god Indra's weapon, the thunderbolt, which symbolises strength. Vajrasana is often called the pelvis posture.

Effect

Vajrasana is primarily a meditation posture, in which it is easy and natural to keep the spine straight, and to breathe calmly and deeply. The posture removes abdominal tension, stimulates blood circulation in the abdomen and facilitates digestion. Vajrasana moderately stretches the muscles of the thighs and shins, makes the ankles and knees supple, and alleviates weariness and soreness in the back. Body energy flows smoothly, calmness and equanimity ensue, and the mind becomes tuned to inner contemplation. Vajrasana is a common meditation posture among Buddhists and Muslims, and many Japanese take their meals sitting in this pose. By sitting in vajrasana for 5-10 minutes after a meal, digestion is stimulated.

In general

When you have sore insteps, let the heels slide out to the sides or sit in variation No. 1, where the feet cross one another. Pains in the knees, calves, ankles and thighs disappear when this posture is practised slowly. You may use leg exercise No. 6 (p. 41). If the soreness continues, sit on a 10-15 cm high stool and tuck your legs under it, or place a pillow between your feet and buttocks. Variations

Technique

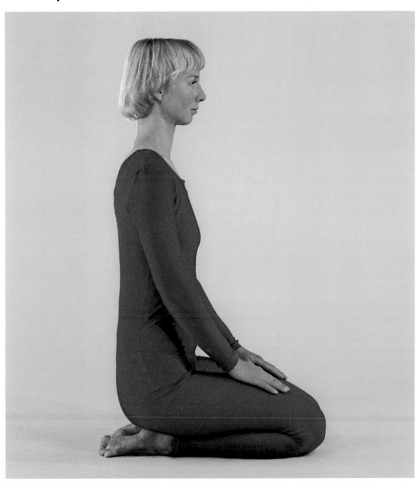

Sit on both heels with knees together, each pelvic bone resting on a heel. Straighten the spine by lifting the breast-bone and the top of the head, chin slightly tucked in. Avoid excessive lumbar curve and keep the shoulders lowered and relaxed.

Nos. 2 and 3 require a great deal of suppleness in the knee joints, and these variations in particular should be practised carefully and slowly. In the beginning sit on a folded blanket, gradually reducing its thickness until you are able to reach the floor without discomfort.

Duration

So long as it is comfortable.

Variations

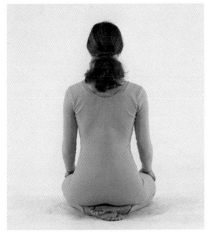

1. Place the right instep in the arch of the left foot. Repeat with the left foot on top.

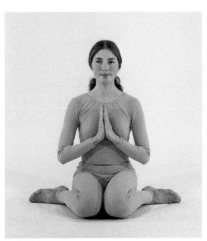

2. Resting both hands on the heels, carefully lower the buttocks between the feet.

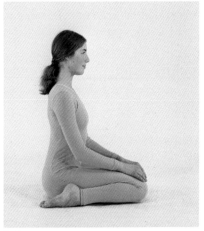

3. The feet may point out to the sides as in No. 2, or backward along the thighs.

Ardha chandrasana

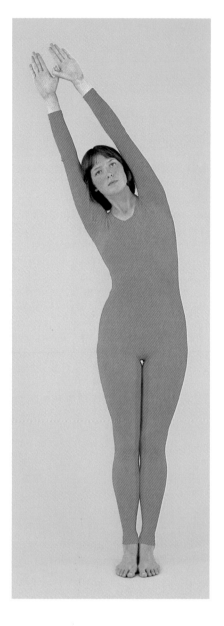

Name

Ardha chandrasana means half-moon posture.

Effect

Ardha chandrasana is a beneficial exercise for the back and is within the scope of most people. It involves a strong stretch and multi-directional movements of the back, which lessen pressure and stimulate metabolism in the vertebral discs. This enables them to retain their elasticity and withstand strain from pressure, tension and lop-sided working positions. Alternating contraction and stretching strengthens and relaxes muscles in the back, abdomen and sides of the body. Stretching the respiratory muscles and expanding the chest stimulate breathing, so the lungs are suitably exercised in this pose. At the different stages of the exercise, the internal organs are beneficially massaged, and the circulation is stimulated by the stretching and contraction of the body. Ardha chandrasana has an immediate refreshing effect.

In general

It must be emphasised that the initial position for all standing exercises should be correct. The back must be straight with a natural curve, the shoulders relaxed and lowered, breast-bone slightly raised and chin drawn in a little. Too great a hollow in the small of the back may be corrected by slightly tightening the muscles of the buttocks. If the exercise leaves you feeling tired or sore in the arms and shoulders, then you may lower the arms between the different phases. If you concentrate on the thoracic vertebrae while stretching to the side, and do not move the waist or the hips, the effect of the exercise on the lungs is increased. Take care that the arms are kept close to the ears and do not lean forward. Keep the thoracic vertebrae slightly bent during the forward position. Every time you straighten the body, stretch further with the help of your arms. The straight stretch is beneficial if you have a tendency for a slipped disc, but avoid bending if the spinal column is weak.

Duration

The exercise may be performed 3-4 times to each side.

Technique

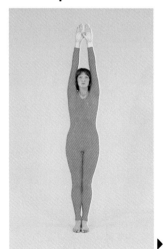

Stand straight with feet together. Tighten the buttocks and stretch both arms overhead, keeping them close to the ears. Turn palms forward and interlock the thumbs.

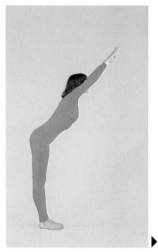

Inhale and stretch right up. Extend the breast-bone while stretching forward, so the body forms a straight line from buttocks to finger-tips. Exhale slowly and come back to vertical.

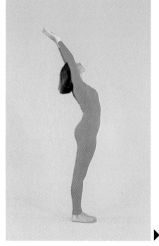

Inhale and stretch right up. Extend breast-bone and tighten the buttocks when bending back in the thoracic vertebrae. Stretch well, exhale and come back to upright.

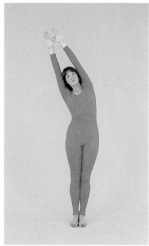

Inhale and stretch straight. Bend to the right in the thoracic vertebrae and exhale, keeping the stretch. Come upright and repeat to the left side. Stretch up straight and lower the arms.

Variation

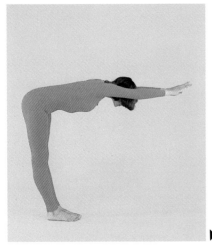

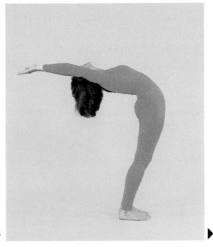

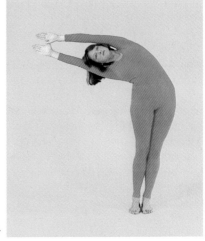

Perform the exercise as described, only bend forward at the hip joint till the body is horizontal.

Arch backward from the waist as far as possible without bending the knees.

Bend over on both sides in turn from the waist without turning the pelvis.

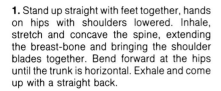

Preliminary exercises

1. Stand up straight with feet together, hands on hips with shoulders lowered. Inhale, stretch and concave the spine, extending the breast-bone and bringing the shoulder blades together. Bend forward at the hips until the trunk is horizontal. Exhale and come up with a straight back.

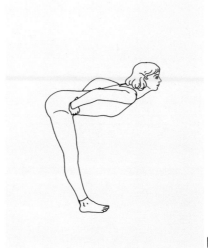

2. Inhale, extend the breast-bone and bring the shoulder blades together. Tighten the buttocks and arch the back without bending at the knees. Carefully curve the neck backwards. Straighten up and exhale.

3. Inhale and bend to the right. Avoid turning the left shoulder or hip forwards. Exhale and relax, thereby reaching further down while lowering the right ear to the right shoulder, face pointing directly forward. Straighten up and inhale. Repeat to the left side.

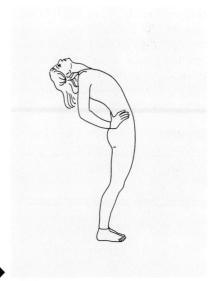

4. Inhale, tighten the buttocks and extend the back. Twist to the right until the chin is above the right shoulder. Avoid twisting the knees. Exhale in the pose. Face forward and repeat to the left.

Finish the series by raising both arms overhead. Inhale, stretch up straight, concave the spine and bend forward at the hips. As far as possible keep the back straight. Finally let arms and head hang forward completely relaxed. Come up slowly, chin tucked in, and inhale.

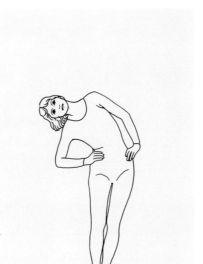

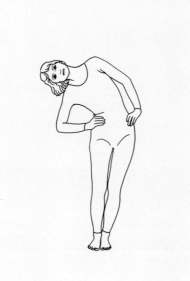

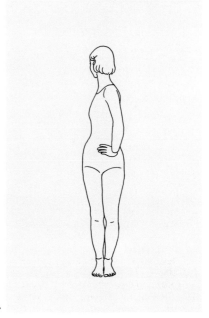

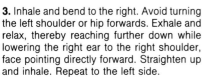

Garudasana

Name

Garuda is a mythological bird.

Effect

Garudasana is a balancing exercise which also strengthens and exercises the leg muscles. It makes the legs, arms, shoulders and hips strong and supple, and releases tension in the shoulders and upper part of the back, especially between the shoulder blades. By stretching the buttocks and thighs it alleviates sciatic and rheumatic pains in the legs.

In general

Garudasana may be prepared for by means of shoulder exercises pp. 30ff., leg and foot exercises (pp. 45ff. as well as the preparatory exercises for vrikshasana (p. 101). First practise the position of the arms, and then that of the legs, perhaps independently. Begin by standing erect, then gradually bend lower as you become accustomed to the posture. Relax the neck and shoulders, keep the back straight and bend at the hips.

Duration

Stand in the pose for a few seconds or for half a minute at the most.

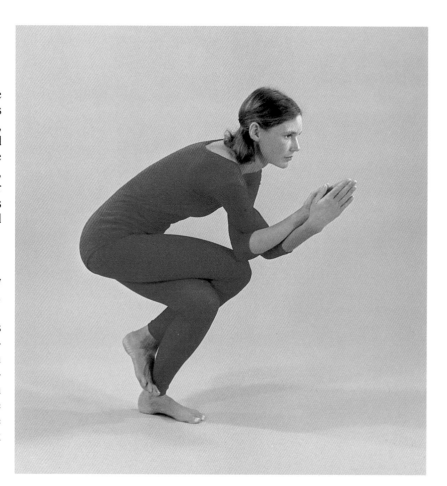

Technique

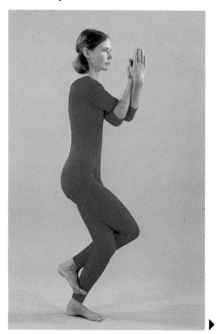

Place the right upper arm in the bend of the left elbow. Twist the right forearm around the left one, joining the palms, thumbs toward the face. Cross the right thigh over the left knee, twist the foot behind the left calf until it rests on the inside of the left ankle.

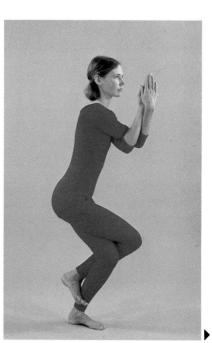

Bend the left knee a little more, keep the back straight, shoulders relaxed. Try to pull the elbows forward, increasing the stretch between the shoulder blades. Look straight forward at the hands.

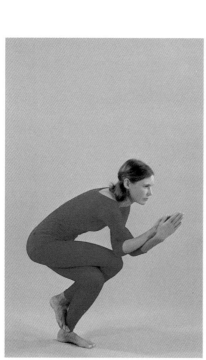

Bend forward and rest the left elbow on the right knee. Breathe slowly and regularly while remaining balanced. Straighten up and carefully relax leg and arm positions. Repeat on the opposite side.

100

Name

Vrikshasana means tree posture.

Effect

In vrikshasana the back and the respiratory muscles are stretched. Therefore the posture helps to overcome tension and weariness in the back and loins; it gives a good stance and promotes deep breathing. The upward stretch stimulates the heart, blood circulation and organs in the upper part of the body, giving the area a slight warmth. The joints of the hips, legs and feet become supple, and the leg muscles are slightly strengthened. This is an effective balancing exercise for counteracting restlessness and nervousness.

In general

In the complete posture take care to ensure that the bent knee is kept straight out to the side, and that the arms do not go forward. It requires a great deal of suppleness to get the foot all the way up to the groin. Until that is achieved, place the foot as far up the thigh as possible. The effect of the posture is increased if you carry out *the complete breath while counting:* for example, inhale calmly for 5 seconds, hold it for 5 seconds and exhale for 5 seconds. Alternatively, use another rhythm which suits your capacity. This breathing should be practised separately, and the muscles should initially become accustomed to the stretching of the posture. It is always a help in balancing postures to relax and concentrate on a balance point, such as an external point at eye level, or a point in the middle of the body at the level of the breast-bone. If you have difficulty in keeping your balance, then practise for a while against a wall or similar support.

Duration

Stand in the posture for half a minute to 1 minute on each leg. The above-mentioned breathing should only be done 3 times.

Technique

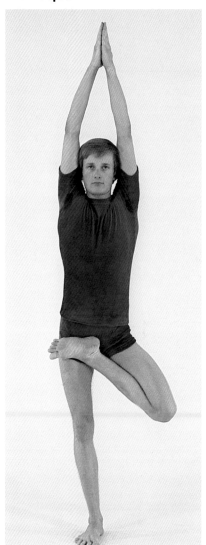

Stand straight with feet parallel and a hip width apart. Bend the left leg and place the foot on the right groin. Turn the bent knee out to the side and pull the buttocks in. Bring the palms together at the chest and stretch upward until the arms are straight and close to the ears. Breathe deeply and regularly. Lower the hands slowly, and hold on to the left knee and foot, while carefully loosening the foot position, then turn the bent knee straight forward and stretch the leg down. Repeat on the other leg.

Variations

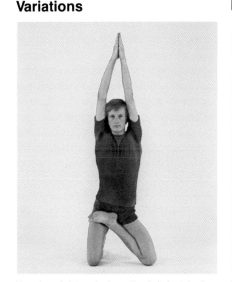

Kneel upright and place the left foot in the right groin. Straighten the back, pulling the buttocks in. Bring the palms together at the chest and stretch them over the head. Lower the hands and carefully relax the leg position.

Preliminary exercises

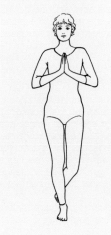

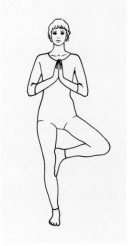

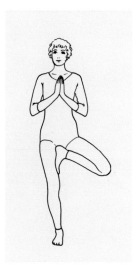

1. Stand erect, feet parallel and slightly apart. Place the left foot behind the right ankle and bring the palms together in front of the chest.

2. Bend the left knee out to the side and slide the sole of the foot up the inside of the right leg. Place the foot at the level of the calf or knee.

3. Bring the foot as high up the thigh as possible. In all the preliminary poses you may stretch up the arms when you are able to keep the balance.

Natarajasana

Name

Nataraja is one of the names of the god Shiva and means the Cosmic Dancer.

Effect

Nataraja is a beautiful balancing posture that gives a natural, straight and graceful stance. It stretches the muscles of the front side of the body and the backs of the knees, making the back and hips supple. The vigorous stretching of the abdominal muscles, together with the bending of the back, is a tonic for the internal organs and aids blood circulation and a sluggish stomach. Stretching the diaphragm and exercising the ribs relax these important respiratory muscles, and therefore the posture benefits incomplete and tense respiration. The exercise makes the shoulder joints supple, alleviating tension pains in the back, neck, shoulders and upper arms.

In general

Natarajasana is not as difficult as it looks, but practice requires concentration on your balancing. In order to practise for the posture you can do the preliminary exercises for dhanurasana (p. 67), to make the back supple. The initial posture must be with straight back, lowered shoulders and legs straight and together. Enter the

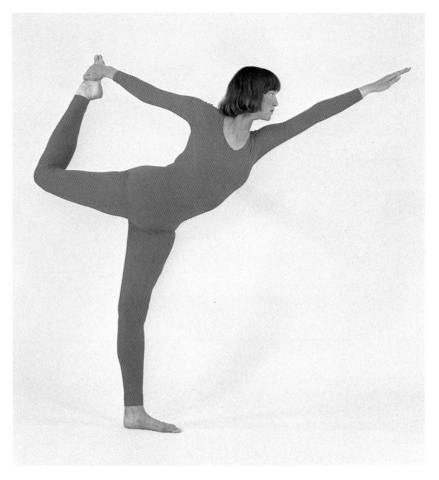

posture slowly and smoothly. Never go so far that you feel pain; if this happens, then lower the raised leg. Stand motionless in the final posture and see that breathing is deep and relaxed. After this exercise you may relax the small of the back in pavanamuktasana (p. 82).

Duration

Remain in the pose for up to half a minute.

Technique

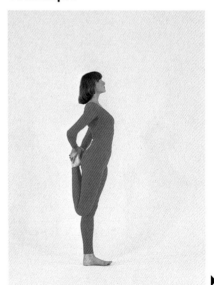

Stand straight, with legs together, shoulders lowered and relaxed. Bend the right leg backward, grasp the foot and pull upward until the knees are together.

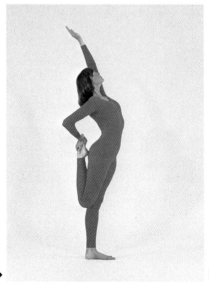

Stretch the left arm upwards, inhale, elongate the spine and arch backward, raising the breast-bone.

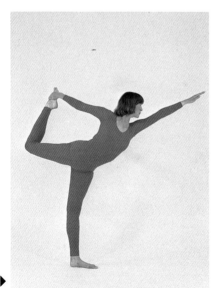

Lean forward with your trunk and left arm, with right hand pulling the right foot upward and exhale. Look at the left hand. Return to upright, lowering the arm and leg. Repeat with the other leg.

Variations

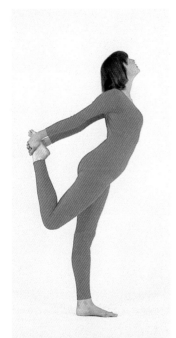

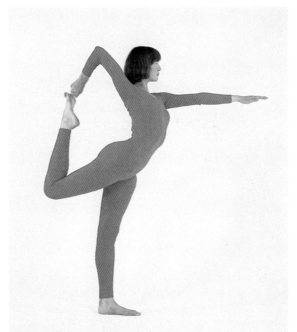

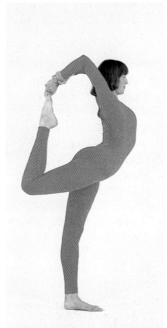

1. Bend the right leg, grasp the foot with both hands and pull backward, extending the breast-bone. Bring the shoulder blades together and arch the whole spine. Repeat with the other leg.

2. Bend the right leg back and grasp the big toe with the right hand. Pull the leg upward, arching the back. Rotate at the shoulder joint, pointing the elbow toward the ceiling. Stretch the left arm forward. Repeat with the other leg.

3. Commence as var. No. 2. Bring the left arm over the head and backward, and grasp the right foot or hand. Repeat with the other leg.

Preliminary exercises

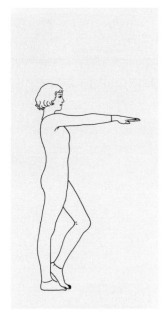

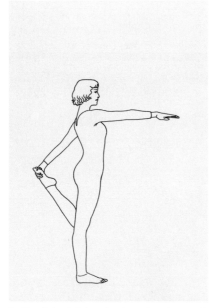

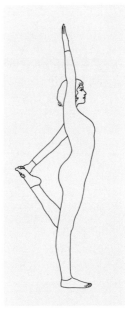

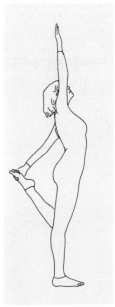

1. Stand with back straight. Bend the left knee forward and place the left foot on the right forefoot with the heel against the right shin. Stretch the right arm forward. Concentrate on a point at eye level.

2. Bend the left foot backward and grasp it with the left hand, keeping the knees close together. Relax the left thigh, keeping the breast-bone raised, shoulders lowered and relaxed.

3. Stretch the right arm toward the ceiling. When you are well balanced you may proceed to No. 4.

4. Arch backward, raising the breast-bone and look upward. Repeat all the preliminary exercises with opposite arm and leg position.

Trikonasana

Name
Trikonasana means triangle posture.

Effect
Trikonasana stretches the spinal column effectively, thus leading to a supple body. It stimulates the spinal nerves and alleviates back pain. The muscles are contracted, stretched and relaxed, which aids respiration, blood circulation and muscular metabolism. The posture stretches the muscles on the inner side of the thighs, hips, ribs and shoulders. It massages the intestines and has an overall purifying effect on the organism.

In general
Take care that the feet are parallel and point straight forward. During the sideways bend the body must not move forward, nor the legs bend. It is easier to keep the hips still if you tighten the buttock muscles slightly. Try to keep the upper arm close to the ear all the time. If you want a quick intense programme with many-sided results, you may combine to advantage the dynamic variation where the back is stretched in different directions with suryanamaskar (p. 116).
Avoid this exercise if there is a tendency for a slipped disc.

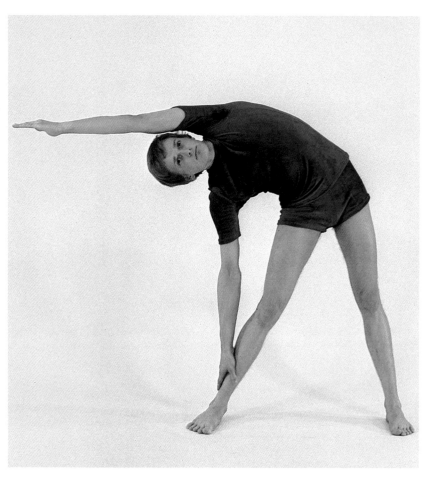

Duration
Stand in the posture for up to 3 minutes, or repeat it at short intervals a couple of times to each side.

Technique

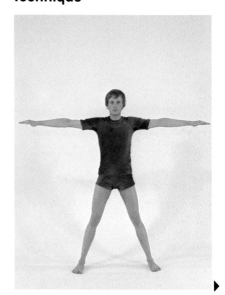

Stand with back straight, feet parallel and about 80 cm apart. Extend the arms horizontally to either side and tighten the buttocks.

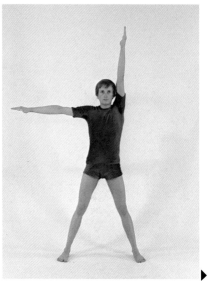

Eliminate excessive lumbar curve. Inhale and turn the left palm up, raising the arm to the left ear. Stretch upward.

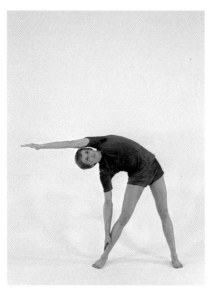

Bend over to the right without turning the trunk, and place the right hand on the lower leg. Exhale and relax going further down. Repeat to the left.

Dynamic variation

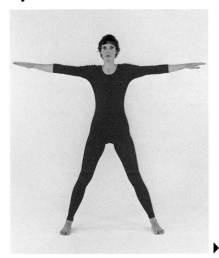
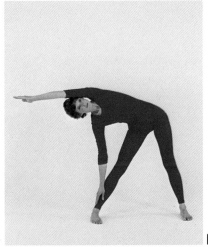
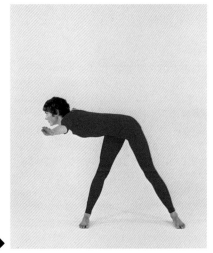

Stand erect with the feet about 80 cm apart and arms horizontal.

Stretch the left arm toward the ceiling and inhale. Bend over to the right and exhale.

Turn the trunk horizontally over the right leg, arms straight out to either side. Stretch the back and inhale.

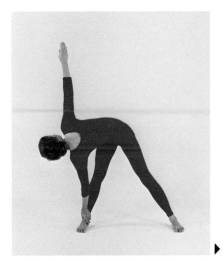
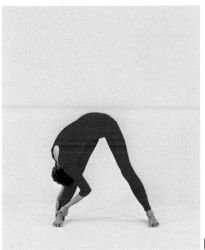
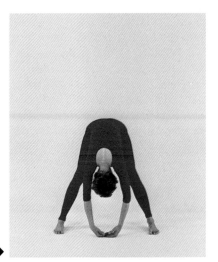

Grasp the right ankle with the left hand and extend the right arm toward the ceiling. Look up and hold the breath.

Lower the right hand to the right ankle. Exhale and pull the trunk toward the leg, keeping the back as straight as possible.

Let trunk, arms and head hang down relaxed between the legs. Come up slowly, chin to chest, and inhale. Repeat to the left.

Preliminary exercises

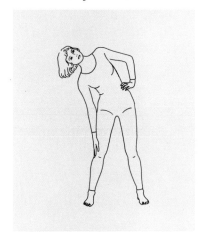
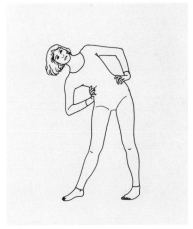
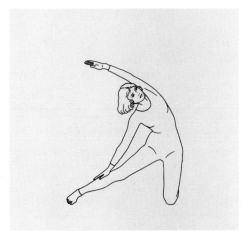

1. Stand with the feet apart at shoulder width and with the back straight. Place the left hand on the left hip. Inhale, elongating the spine, tighten the buttocks and bend over to the right. Repeat to the left.

2. Stand with feet apart, hands on hips, the right foot pointing to the right at 90°, and the left foot at 45°. Inhale, extending the back, push the left hip outward, bend the trunk over to the right and exhale. Repeat opposite.

3. Kneel upright, extend the right leg sideways with the foot pointing forwards. Place the right hand on the right leg and stretch the left arm up. Inhale, stretch up and bend over the right leg, exhaling. Come up and repeat to the left.

Utkanasana

Name

Utkata means forceful. It is often called the chair.

Effect

Utkatasana is one of the most effective strengthening exercises for the muscles of the feet, calves and thighs. It keeps the knees and ankles supple, stimulates circulation in the legs and feet, and alleviates soreness of the feet. Therefore, it is particularly beneficial for all people whose working posture is standing. This exercise is useful in developing a good lifting technique, and erect posture; it also improves balance and concentration.

In general

During the complete exercise, take care that the heels and knees remain together, and that the weight of the body rests on the toes. When you have achieved balance in the posture, the effect may be increased by stretching the arms over the head with palms together. This variation stretches the abdominal muscles, lifts the diaphragm and stimulates the heart and blood circulation in the upper part of the body. Those with weak legs may support the extended arms on the back of a chair, and only bend the legs as much as they can.

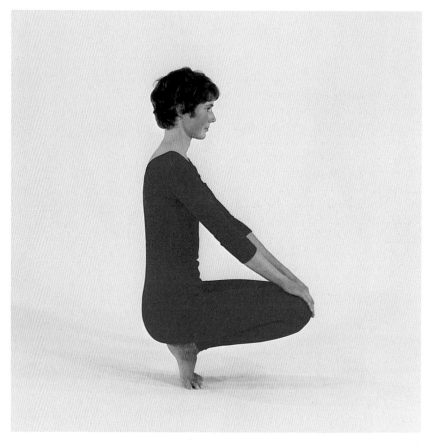

Avoid straining so much that you are short of breath and get heart palpitations. When the ankles are weak or there are varicose veins, the soles of the feet may be kept on the floor; alternatively, a book or similar support can be placed under the heels.

Duration

Repeat the exercise a couple of times, or remain in it from half a minute to 1 minute. Avoid straining.

Technique

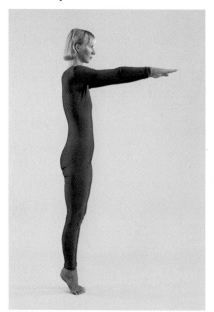

Stand up straight, feet together, arms horizontally stretched forward. Concentrate on a fixed point during the whole exercise. Come up to stand on the toes.

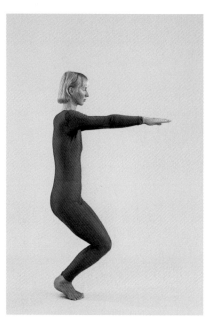

Inhale, tighten the buttocks, aligning the back, and push both knees forward while lowering the trunk directly over the heels. Keep the knees and heels together.

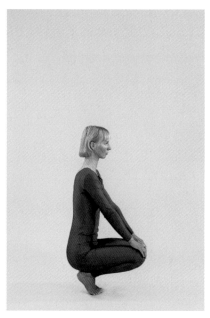

Exhale, resting on the heels. Stay with the back straight, hands resting on the knees, and breathe quietly. Inhale and come up in the same way. Exhale lowering the heels and arms.

Name

Bhadrasana means the good or noble posture.

Effect

Bhadrasana stretches the muscles and tendons of the inner side of the thigh. It makes the hip and knee joints supple and is therefore a good preliminary exercise to padmasana and the other meditation postures. Bhadrasana allays tension states in the pelvic floor and abdominal organs, and may help to cure venous stasis in the abdomen and also haemorrhoids. It is one of the few yoga postures that are recommended during pregnancy. If one can keep the back straight, it is a good posture for pain in the loins and sciatica. Advanced yogis use a variation of the posture, mulabandhasana (var. No. 2), in connection with certain breathing exercises.

In general

In the beginning most people find that they cannot get their knees close to the floor. This is normal and should not cause discouragement. If one tries to relax and give way with the legs, the knees will gradually come down by themselves without any effort. It is important to keep the back straight during this exercise. It is tempting to bend the body in order to lessen the stretching effect on the thighs, but if this is done, the effect is diminished and tension arises in the small of the back, together with a strain on the vertebrae and pressure

Technique

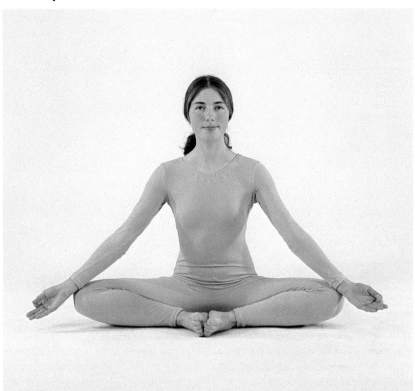

Sit with a straight back. Pull the feet close in to the crutch and lower the knees to the sides, keeping the soles of the feet together. Grasp the feet and straighten up the back by raising the breast-bone. Relax in the hip joints and the inside of the thighs, lowering the knees to the floor. When it is possible to remain with a straight back, the hands can rest on the knees.

on the internal organs. If support is necessary, sit with the buttocks against a wall. In the correct posture the heels are close to the body, the legs rest on the floor from ankle to hip, and the back is straight. Be careful when coming out of the posture. Grasp the knees and pull them together in front of the chest. Slowly stretch the legs out in front. As a counter-exercise, sit for a while in vajrasana (p. 97), possibly with the buttocks between the legs.

Duration

Sit as long as it is comfortable. Use the time to do a concentration exercise; concentrate on either an external visible object or on the breathing.

Variations

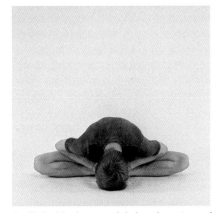

1. Sit in bhadrasana. Inhale, elongate and concave the spine. Exhale, pulling in the abdomen, and bend pelvis and trunk forward to rest the forehead on the floor. Come up with a straight back.

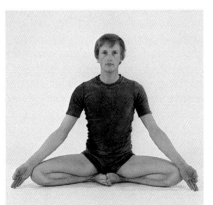

2. Place the hands on the floor and lift the buttocks to rest on the heels. This variation demands considerable flexibility in the ankles.

Preliminary exercise

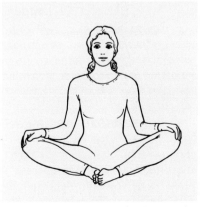

Sit erect, bring the soles of the feet together and pull the heels closer. Extend the spine and relax hips and knees, allowing the legs to sink toward the floor by themselves.

Savasana

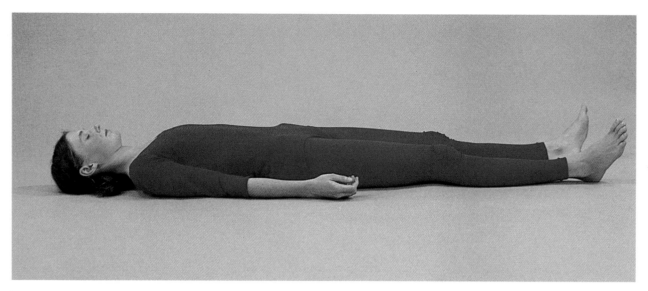

Name

Savasana means corpse pose.

Effects

Savasana works deeply on both body and mind, reduces all kinds of tensions and gives rest and relaxation. It combats mental troubles and worries, clears the mind and calms the emotions. Savasana also helps the nerve energy to circulate evenly throughout the body, thereby improving the general state of health. It reduces any kind of pain and brings a smooth flow to the heart and respiration. When you become familiar with the exercise, you will experience an inner peace which influences daily life and makes you a more harmonious and balanced person.

In general

Initially, learn the physical posture as described under technique, and make sure that the central axis of the body is straight. If you have any pain in the back of the neck, it may help to use a small cushion. If your back is too curved, you can also use a cushion under the lumbar spine. When the body is comfortably placed in this posture you can begin with deeper physical relaxation.

Close the eyes and try to be aware of the whole body as an entity. Notice if there are any restless or disturbed areas and try to calm them mentally. Be aware of your breathing and do some rounds of the complete yogic breath (p. 126), until you have removed all respiratory tension. Make sure that the breath is flowing in a slow, even rhythm of its own, and do not try to influence it further, but forget it. Now feel the heaviness of the body as it is lying prone on the floor. Notice a mild warmth all over that makes it soft and pleasant.

Then begin a deep relaxation of the body from the feet upwards. Imagine how you withdraw all tensions from the right foot and then from the left foot. Continue mentally to relax the lower legs, the hamstring muscles, knees and thighs, ending up with the hips. Let there be no tension or active awareness left in the legs. Leave them completely to themselves and forget them. Now continue by withdrawing all tension from the pelvic region. Relax the anus, buttocks and abdominal muscles. Feel how the whole area collapses, as it were, and withdraw your attention from it. Continue the process and relax the back from the loins upward to the shoulders, observing how it makes the body sink further down on the floor. Next, turn to the front part of the body, and make sure that when your attention moves upward, no tension is left in the chest and the whole trunk is totally relaxed. Forget it! Now turn to the arms. Begin with the fingers and hand of the right arm and proceed upward to the shoulder. Do the same with the left. Then relax the throat in a gliding movement ending with the tongue and mouth. Loosen the jaws, chin and facial muscles. Relax the eyes and temples, completing the process with the forehead and scalp. Now your body is in a state of deep relaxation and lies passively as a corpse. Do not let your attention focus on it and do not try to feel anything physically, and forget the outer world completely. When the body and senses have been made to relax, you are left experiencing your own mental activity. During this stage you will notice innumerable thoughts flowing through the mind. Just let them come and go. Do not pay any attention to them but remain as a passive witness. Ignore this profuse activity and try to feel an all-pervading silence into which everything gets absorbed. Focus your whole attention on this perfect, undisturbed state of peace and try to let it fill your whole being.

If you find it too difficult to transcend all disturbing thoughts, it may be helpful to calm the mind by visualising some attractive and peaceful scenery, such as a vast expanse of the ocean or a clear blue sky. Alternatively, you may find it easy to imagine the great stillness of deep, infinite space. Whatever you choose, try to concentrate the mind completely and become absorbed in a state of peace. If you practise regularly, this process will have an invigorating effect on your whole being.

When the exercise is over, take some deep breaths and stretch the body thoroughly, then open the eyes and sit for a few moments before rising.

Duration

Savasana should always be the last exercise, in which one usually spends some 10 to 15 minutes.

Technique

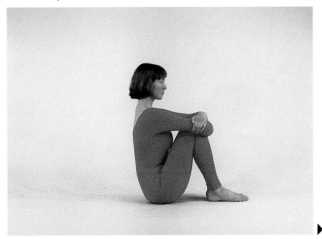

Sit up straight with knees held close to the body, so that the legs, chin and nose are aligned with the central axis of the body.

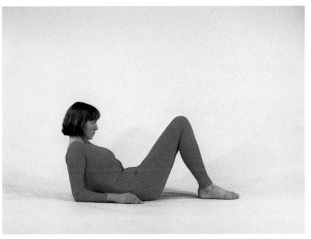

Place the palms on the floor beside the buttocks and relax while bending backwards. Rest on the forearms while slowly rolling the lower spine down on the floor.

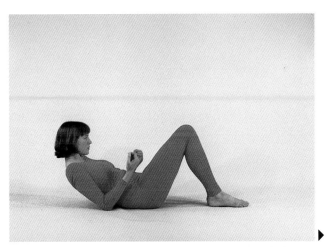

Rest on the elbows while lowering the thoracic and cervical vertebrae one by one. The head and spine should form a straight line, and the weight of the body should be distributed equally on each side.

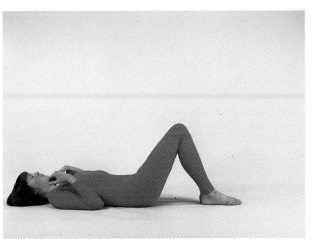

Stretch the neck and tuck the chin in slightly while keeping the head erect. Bend the forearms, touching the shoulders with the fingertips, and pull the elbows downward.

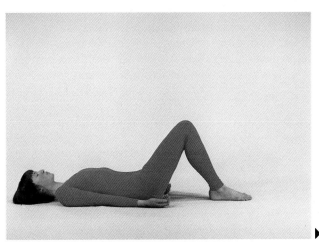

Lower the forearms to the floor with palms up, relaxing the arms and shoulders. Slide the heels along the floor until the legs are straight, then relax the legs and feet.

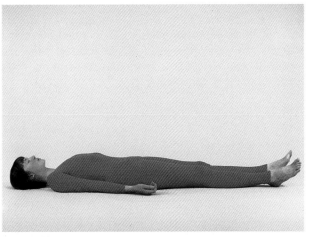

Now, the body should lie full length, the central axis forming a straight line. Lie with eyes softly shut and with a feeling of deep relaxation in body and mind.

Meditation postures

The Indian yogi Swami Narayanananda describes meditation as an "unbroken concentration of the mind on one point at will". Meditation is an effective means of gaining peace of mind, awakening the latent creative Power or the Kundalini Shakti, and reaching a higher stage of spiritual development. It is the most important discipline of yoga, and the means used by yogis to attain the highest goal, namely, Freedom (Moksha) or Cosmic Consciousness. Usually the mind is scattered and constantly externalised through the sense organs, the body is restless and breathing and rhythm of the organs irregular. In this state the life force is scattered in all directions; one gets tired and has to recoup this lost energy through rest and sleep. In meditation, however, all the scattered forces of the mind are gathered at a concentrated mental point, as the body is put in a motionless posture which allows its energy to flow towards the object of meditation. The process implies that body and mind are composed, while at the same time a strong recharging of energy takes place.

So in order to be able to meditate, it is necessary to put the body in a posture in which you may sit immobile for a considerable time without becoming tired or falling asleep, and in which it is quite possible to shut out awareness of the body.

Padmasana (the lotus posture) is the most important of all meditation postures; in addition, there are a number of other postures, mostly variations of this with the legs in various cross-legged positions.

Meditation postures usually require practice to make the legs supple, especially the knee joints. For this purpose the preliminary series for padmasana may be used (see page 113). It is important to be very careful with these exercises in order to avoid injury to the knees. In particular, it is risky to force the legs into a posture if the knees are cold. Begin with a couple of warm-up exercises, massaging the knees until they are warm, then slowly and carefully bring the legs into the posture. If shooting pains are felt, you must immediately relax or discontinue it.

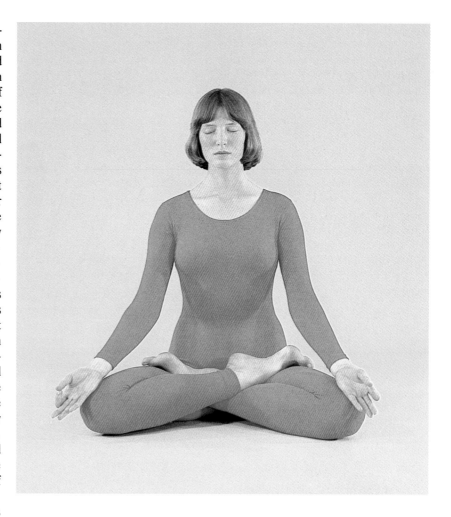

A meditation posture must be firm and stable and the body should not shake or sway. Therefore it is preferable to have both knees on the floor, so that there is a broad supporting surface. Another important point is that the middle axis of the body must be quite straight. You should not bend to either side, or forwards or backwards. This leads to strain, tension, pain and tiredness, which will disturb you and make meditation impossible. In a correct meditation posture, the back, neck and head must be in a straight line; that is, if you imagine a vertical line drawn from the top of the head to the abdomen, it would hit a point in the perineum, between the anus and the genitals. Straighten the back, keep the chest a little forward, lower the shoulders and draw the shoulder blades slightly backwards. Lift the head and draw in the chin a little, so that a small contraction of the throat is achieved. Likewise contract the anus slightly, and pull the buttocks a little backwards and upwards. This

will make it possible to keep a straight posture for a long time without tiring. At the same time the resulting stretch of the abdomen and raised diaphragm almost automatically lead to deeper and easier breathing. If you sit in a bent posture, breathing becomes shallow and strained, digestion and circulation of the blood are impaired and back pains occur. Furthermore, if you try to meditate in a posture with a bent back, you will discover it is very difficult to achieve mind-control. This is due to the fact that a bent posture inhibits the subtle nerve currents which are connected with thought functions. In such a position, single-minded concentration is prevented, as breathing becomes short and strained, and restlessness and discomfort are experienced.

The place where you sit in a meditation posture should be neither too soft nor too hard. A folded blanket will do. When you sit in the posture, take care to avoid draughts and cold. During meditation and pranayama exercises (see page 129), the organism becomes sensitive and easily absorbs cold. Pay special attention to protecting the neck area and the knee joints, which are sensitive parts of the body. If you have difficulty in keeping the back straight in the posture, it may help to put a small pillow or something similar under the buttocks, but let this support be as small as possible.

When you have chosen a suitable posture, you should stick to it and practise it regularly every day. Only gradually and slowly should you increase the duration. When knee pains increase, you should not suddenly break off the posture, instead, ease off very slowly and stretch or relax the legs briefly, before continuing in the posture.

There is no time limit for the meditation postures. The longer you can sit, the better. The great yogis of the past and present have sat in these postures for 10-15 hours without difficulty, or continuously for days without the least physical discomfort; on the contrary in doing so, they have experienced the highest bliss. This is mentioned, not to encourage readers to try something similar, which is sure to cause disorders, but to let them know that such a thing is possible. In order to be able to sit for a very long time, it is necessary to be capable of engaging the mind in concentration on the object of meditation for hours at a time, without being distracted by the body or anything else. In general, you will find it beneficial to practise sitting motionless in a meditation posture for half an hour continuously.

It is outside the scope of this book to describe the actual meditation technique. Meditation is a personal affair which should be learned individually from an experienced teacher, who through it has reached the aspired-after goal. Interested readers are referred to Swami Narayanananda's *The Secrets of Mind-Control,* in which a simple and concise introduction to the subject is given.

Technique

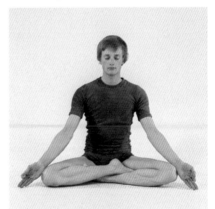

Svastikasana (the auspicious pose). Bend the left leg and place foot close to the right groin. Bend the right leg and place the heel in the left groin, tucking in the toes between the left thigh and calf. Pull the front part of the left foot up between the right thigh and calf, thereby locking the leg position. Straighten the back.

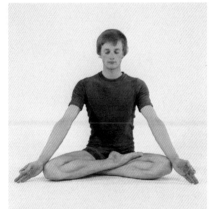

Ardha padmasana (half lotus pose). Bend the left leg and place the foot close to the groin, the sole of the foot resting along the right thigh. Bend the right leg, grasp the foot and turn the sole upward, placing the instep on the left thigh close to the groin. Lower the knee toward the floor and straighten up the back. Perform the pose with the other leg on top.

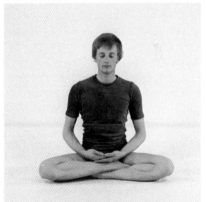

Siddhasana (the accomplished pose): this pose is only suitable for men. Bend the left leg and press the heel against the perineum, with the sole along the right thigh. Bend the right leg and place the heel at the pubic bone above the genitals, which should not be pressed. Place the front part of the foot between the left thigh and calf. Sit straight and apply mula bandha (p. 120).

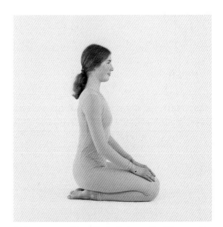

Vajrasana (thunderbolt pose). Sit on the heels with knees together and the pelvic bones resting directly on each heel. As a variation, slide the heels outward and rest the buttocks between the heels, big toes remaining together. Sit erect with hands resting on thighs.

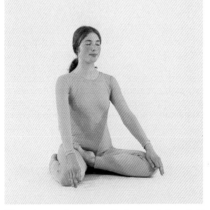

Veerasana (hero pose). Bend at the right knee and place the foot along the right hip. Bend the left leg, turn the sole upward and place the instep on the right thigh close to the groin. Both pelvic bones should rest equally on the floor to keep the spine erect.

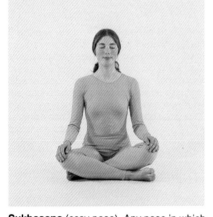

Sukhasana (easy pose). Any pose in which it is possible to sit comfortably with a straight back, e.g. the simple cross-legged posture, resting each knee on the opposite foot. Or place the right foot on the floor close to the crutch and the left foot close in front with both shins resting on the floor.

Padmasana

Name

Padmasana means lotus posture. The lotus flower symbolises pure Consciousness.

Effect

Padmasana is the most famous of all the yoga asanas. It is the best meditation posture, because it creates harmony, peace and balance in the whole organism, making it possible to sit unmoving for a long time in meditative concentration, without being disturbed by physical sensations. It weakens the firm hold the sense-organs have on the body, calms the emotions, and so helps to tune the mind to inner contemplation. Padmasana leads to deep, calm and smoothly flowing respiration, and is the preferred posture for breathing exercises (pranayama). It strengthens the abdomen, counteracts high blood pressure and creates supple hips and legs. It has a very stimulating effect on the nervous system and alleviates physical and mental tiredness.

In general

The posture should be practised slowly and carefully. Avoid straining the legs immediately before or after doing it. Slowly take the legs into the position and never do it if your knees are cold. As you come out of the posture, grasp your feet with your hands and carefully place them on the floor.

Technique

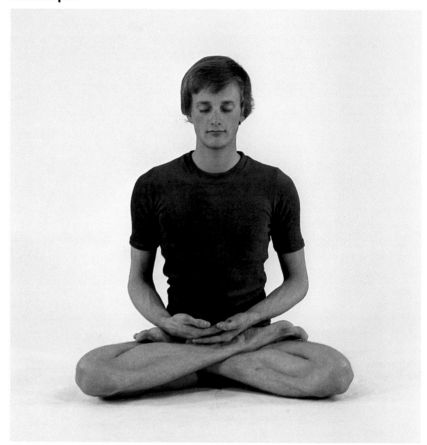

Sit erect with legs in front. Bend one leg, take hold of the foot, turning the sole upward and place the instep at the opposite groin. Bend the other leg and place the foot correspondingly in the other groin, so that the ankles are crossed and the feet close to the hip bones. Place the left hand on the heels, palm upward, and rest the right hand in the left one. Keep the back and neck straight, shoulders lowered, with knees resting on the floor.

Then lift both knees up towards the chest, straighten the feet and slowly stretch the legs in front of you. Take care to keep your legs together when you stand up, so that they are evenly stretched. Avoid getting up before you feel normal strength in the knee joints. This applies to all meditation postures.

Variations

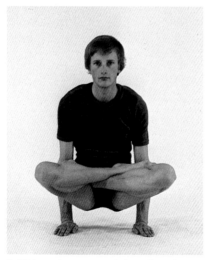

1. Sit in padmasana, and place the palms on the floor beside the hips. Inhale, hold the breath and lift the trunk, balancing on the hands. Lower quietly and exhale.

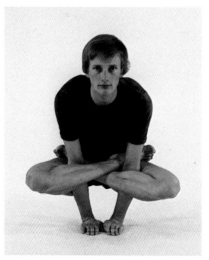

2. Sit in padmasana. Bring the arms down between the calves, thighs and feet, and place the palms on the floor. Inhale and raise the trunk. Lower and exhale.

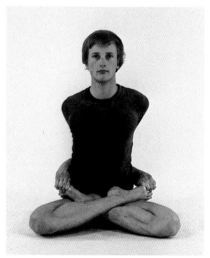

3. Sit in padmasana. Move the feet closer to the hip bones. Pull the shoulders back and cross the arms behind the back to grasp the big toes. Tuck in the chin.

112

Preliminary exercises

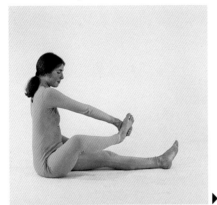

Sit erect with legs in front. Bend the right knee and catch hold of the arch with the right hand. Turn the sole toward the body and push the knee to the right side.

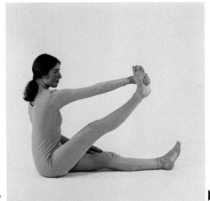

Stretch the right leg upward and outward, still turning the sole upward. Keep the back straight.

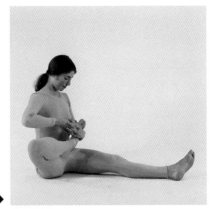

Place the right foot on the left wrist and lock the fingers. Keeping the foot close to the trunk, cautiously move the leg to the right and left alternately.

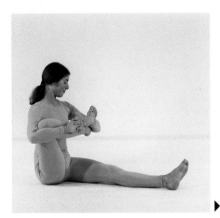

Place the foot in the bend of the elbow, bring the right arm round the knee and interlock the fingers. Pull the leg toward the body and move it carefully to the left and right alternately.

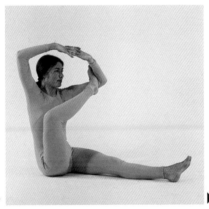

Raise the arms to pull the leg upward, raising it as high as possible without bending the back.

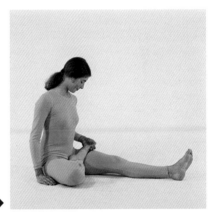

Lower the heel to the navel. Place the instep on the left thigh close to the groin, turning the sole up, and lower the knee to the floor. Hold the knee, bending it to the chest, and extend the leg straight forward.

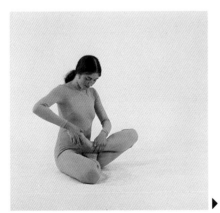

Repeat the preliminary exercise with the other leg. Cautiously try to place each foot in the opposite groin, alternately with the right leg and then the left leg on top.

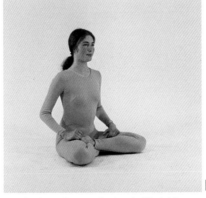

Pull the feet close to the trunk. Straighten up the back extending the breast-bone, and lower the shoulders. Tuck in the chin, slightly elongating the neck.

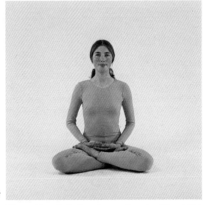

Place the left hand on the heels, palm upward, and rest the right hand in the left one. Maintain the pose, keeping as relaxed as possible and concentrate on breathing deeply and regularly.

Yoga mudra

Name

Yoga means union, and *mudra* is a seal, which also signifies a closed circuit.

Effect

This posture is an asana as well as a mudra. It has a powerful stretching effect on the muscles in the arms, shoulders, back, loins, buttocks and legs. The posture is thus an effective cure for overall tension. It is especially effective for tiredness and stiffness in the loins and is used by many to arouse the body after meditation. It stimulates blood supply in the back, the upper part of the body and the head, and massages the abdominal organs. This exercise helps to cure constipation and a sluggish stomach, and pressure from the heels strongly stimulates the digestive tract. The variation with hands on the heels increases the pressure and acts as an additional tonic; further, it is recommended as a practice for the improvement of slack, descended abdominal organs. Yoga mudra also has a calming effect on excited emotions and makes you feel you have received a burst of energy.

In general

The posture presupposes you have mastered padmasana (page 112) and are supple in the back and hip joints. Even then it may be difficult to do the full forward bend that should mainly

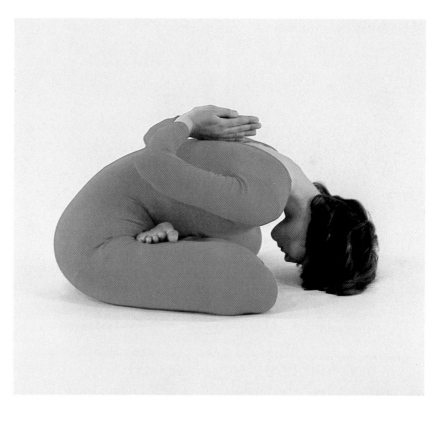

take place from the hips. You can either use some of the preliminary exercises, or bend as far forward as possible, staying there and trying to relax. This will automatically bring you closer to the posture and give speedy results. Be careful if you have a hernia of the groin or a tendency towards slipped disc in the small of the back.

Duration

Yoga mudra may be performed with bahya kumbhaka (external suspension) 3 or 4 times, inhaling and exhaling between every round; or you may stay in the posture breathing normally for a couple of minutes. The variation with the hands on the heels must not be done for more than a few seconds.

Technique

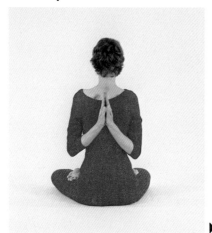

Sit in padmasana (o. 112). Let the finger-tips meet behind the lower back and bring the palms together moving the hands up between the shoulder blades.

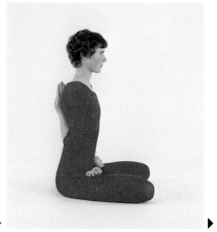

Inhale and extend the spine raising the breast-bone. Lower the shoulders backward and elongate the neck.

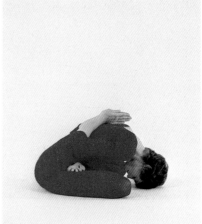

Exhale, pull the abdomen in and bend forward to rest the top of the head on the floor. Relax breathing quietly. Carefully unbend the back and slide the hands down.

Variations

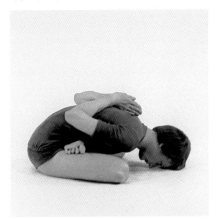

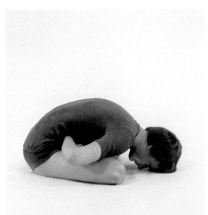

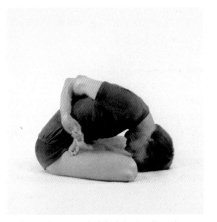

1. Perform yoga mudra with the forehead on the floor as far from the knees as possible. Raise the head, inhale, bring the shoulder blades together and come up with a straight back.

2. Place the hands on heels and perform yoga mudra as described.

3. Cross the arms behind the back and grasp the big toes. Exhale, bending forward to rest the top of the head on the floor.

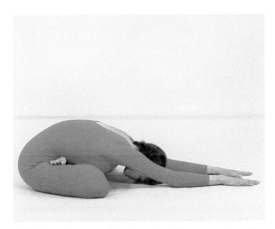

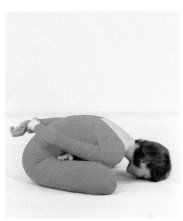

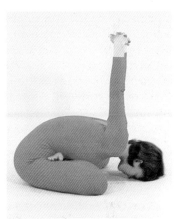

4. Sit in padmasana. Inhale, extend the arms above the head and concave the spine. Exhale and bend forward with a straight back until the arms and forehead rest on the floor.

5. Perform yoga mudra as described, holding the left wrist with the right hand.

6. Sit in padmasana, fingers interlocked behind the back. Inhale, pull the shoulders down extending the breast-bone. Exhale, bend forward and rest the forehead on the floor. Inhale, raising the arms, and lower them exhaling. Inhale, pull back the shoulders and come up with a straight spine.

Preliminary exercises

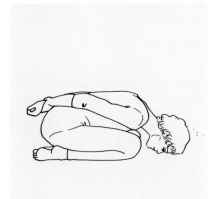

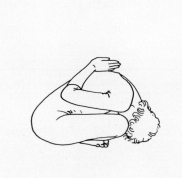

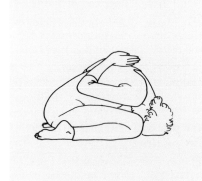

1. Sit in vajrasana (p. 97) and hold the left wrist with the right hand. Inhale, extending the spine. Exhale, bending forward till the forehead or the top of the head rests on the floor. Relax.

2. Sit cross-legged with palms together between the shoulder blades. Bend forward as described, allowing the head to sink towards the floor. Relax in the hips.

3. Sit in vajrasana with buttocks between the feet, and bend forward as described. The hand positions shown can be used with any of the leg positions.

Suryanamaskar

Name

Suryanamaskar means a salute to the sun.

Effect

Suryanamaskar is a series of 12 postures which provide the individual with a highly beneficial all-round exercise within a short space of time. Alternating stretching and bending acts as a "pump" in the sluggish areas of the legs, back and abdomen, leading to deeper breathing and improvement in blood circulation. Gentle and effective stimulation is a result of the activity of muscles in the arms and legs, together with massaging and stretching of the abdominal organs. In these exercises the muscle movements, body postures and breathing are co-ordinated in a way that facilitates a rhythmical balance among the different organs of the body. Suryanamaskar overcomes stiffness and sluggishness and has a refreshing, invigorating effect on both mind and body. After a couple of rounds you feel alert and fit, and there is no better way to start the day than by doing this exercise. If you cannot spare the time for an extensive yoga programme, suryanamaskar is a good alternative. The series can also be used as a warm-up routine before regular yoga asanas or sport.

In general

This exercise was originally meant to be performed at sunrise while facing the east and reciting auspicious mantras, as a kind of reverent salute or tribute to the sun and its life-giving light. The yogis consider that the first activities and impressions of the day relate to how you feel for the rest of the day. When you do suryanamaskar and reflect on the all-pervading light, you create a good and positive foundation for the day's activities.

The 12 postures in suryanamaskar must be done calmly, evenly and rhythmically, avoiding sudden jerks, interruptions or a change of tempo. Find a rhythm that suits you. The most important thing is that the exercises are performed in an easy, relaxed manner.

If you become tired or breathless, you may either have done the exercise too quickly or repeated it too many times. It may be a help in the beginning to learn the series without concerning yourself with the breathing; however, follow the recommended breathing as soon as the postures are mastered. In positions Nos. 3 and 11 the palms must be on the floor – if you cannot do this without bending your legs, you can bend them in order to reach the floor. When the palms are down, they must remain in the same place and not be moved until you straighten up again. If necessary, where wrists are weak, you may point the finger-tips outwards. In positions Nos. 6, 7 and 8, the toes must remain on the same spot. If you find it impossible to lower the heels in the 9th position, you can move the feet a step forward. In the 6th position you can first lower the knees, then the chest and forehead, until you are strong enough to lower all three points simultaneously. Always begin by bending first the right knee and then the left, as this has an important effect on digestion. If you only do the series once, you can bend the right leg first (No. 4) and then the left (No. 10).

Avoid bending the spinal column if you are prone to slipped discs; instead bend the legs in the 3rd and 11th positions. If you have weak hip or knee joints, you must adapt the postures accordingly. Be careful also if there is raised blood pressure.

Duration

Begin by performing suryanamaskar once only, and gradually increase the number of times as you feel inclined. Yogis often repeat the series 9 times.

Technique

1. Stand with a straight back and feet together. Press the palms together in front of the chest with forearms horizontal and shoulders relaxed.

2. Inhale, raising the arms over the head. Stretch straight up, tighten the buttocks and lean backward extending the breast-bone and keeping head and arms together.

3. Still stretching the spine, bend forward from the hips exhaling. Place the palms on the floor beside the feet and the forehead on the knees.

4. Take the left leg as far back as possible, and place toes and knee on the floor while bending the right knee, keeping the right heel on the floor. Look up, concaving the spine, and inhale.

5. Keep the weight on the arms, stretch the left knee and extend the right leg beside the left one, so that legs, trunk and head form a straight line.

6. Bend the arms and place forehead, chest and knees on the floor simultaneously. The buttocks are slightly raised and the elbows close to the trunk. Exhale and pull the abdomen in.

7. Extend the arms, arching the spine backward without lifting the thighs off the floor. Lower the shoulders, bend the head back and inhale.

8. Lift the buttocks high, stretching the legs, so that the weight rests on toes and palms and the head is in between the arms. Hold the breath.

9. Transfer the weight backward, lowering the heels. Straighten out the shoulder joints and back, bend the chin to the chest and exhale.

10. Bring the right foot forward and place the whole sole of the foot on the floor between the hands and lower the left knee. Concave the spine, look up and inhale.

11. Bring the left foot forward beside the right one extending the legs. Bend the forehead toward the knee and exhale.

12. Uncoil the spine. Raise the arms, stretch and arch slightly backward while inhaling. Straighten up, join the palms together at the chest and exhale. Repeat the whole series bending the other leg.

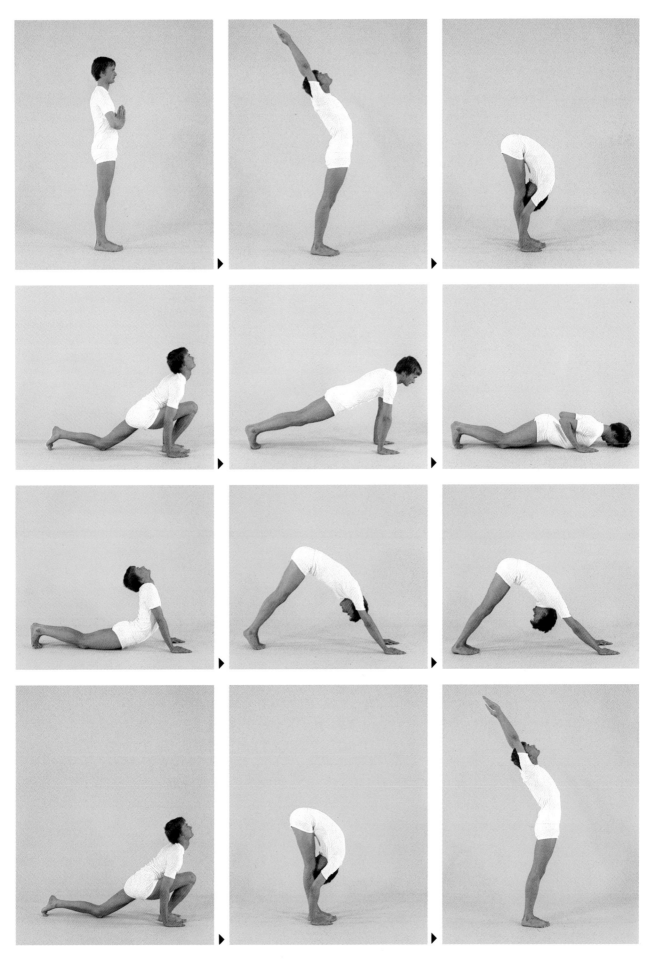

Chapter 3
Mudras and bandhas

Mudras and *bandhas* are the names of a small group of important yoga exercises. A *mudra* is a seal, and *bandha* is a lock. These "bindings" are exercises where a local muscle area is either contracted or subjected to pressure, with the aim of controlling the subtle nerve energy, or *prana* (see glossary, p. 158). As a result it is possible to influence the direction of the prana currents, thus gaining control over the vital forces.

On the spiritual plane these exercises are done to awaken the latent spiritual energy, or Kundalini Shakti, which is the central power embracing all powers. If the exercises are done for this purpose, you must practise meditation regularly, do pranayama and follow the way of life advocated by yoga.

The mudras and bandhas are especially concentrated in the neck area (*jalandhara bandha*), the abdominal area (*uddiyana bandha*), and the anus area (*mula bandha*). They are performed either one at a time or in combination, and they often constitute part of an asana or breathing exercise.

Jalandhara bandha

Name

Jala denotes the network of nerves or nadis that conduct the nerve currents through the neck and throat area, and *bandha* means to lock these.

Effect

This bandha is usually done in connection with breath retention (kumbhaka) in pranayama. It counteracts the pressure in the ears, eyes and head, which arises by holding the breath with full lungs and raised abdomen (antara kumbhaka with uddiyana bandha). Jalandhara bandha helps to ensure that the energy created by the breathing exercises can be controlled and led through the right channels. It also has a calming effect on the incessant automatic thought currents, which prevent real inner peace and drain the mind of energy.

While the breath is held the frequency of the heart-beat will rise, but when you do jalandhara bandha, a reflex is triggered that makes the heart beat normally and calmly. The forward bend also entails a stretching of the cervical vertebrae and whole spinal column, which may alleviate various painful states.

In general

Jalandhara bandha can be practised in connection with sarvangasana (p. 54) and halasana (p. 58), as in these postures you automatically perform this bandha. If you do jalandhara bandha in connection with uddiyana bandha (p. 121), you must always completely exhale and do jalandhara before drawing up the abdomen with lungs empty.

Duration

As long as you can hold the breath.

Technique

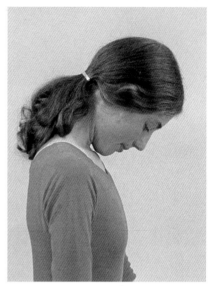

Inhale, contract the muscles of the throat, closing the air-pipe by drawing the tongue slightly backward and up. Stretch the neck and bend it forward pressing the chin against the breast-bone, without bending in the thoracic vertebrae. Lift the head, relax the throat and exhale. The bandha can also be applied between exhalation and inhalation.

Mula bandha

Name

Mula means root or source, and in particular the area around anus.

Effect

Mula bandha is a contractive exercise that locks the sphincters in the anus and draws in the perineum between the anus and the genitals. This bandha influences and helps to control the nervous activity at the floor of the pelvis and the root (mula) of the spinal column. Mula bandha stimulates this area, and leads the subtle nerve currents (prana) upwards, which helps to vitalise the organism. This bandha counteracts haemorrhoids and irritation of the genitals; it also stimulates digestion and blood circulation in the abdomen. Mula bandha is usually performed together with uddiyana bandha (p. 121) and jalandhara bandha (p. 120).

In general

Mula bandha is mostly done in connection with pranayama and certain asanas such as shirsasana, viparita karani, halasana, paschimottanasana and ustrasana.

Duration

This depends on the duration of the aforementioned exercises of which it is part. If the contraction is kept up for too long, it may lead to constipation.

Technique

Mula bandha is generally performed sitting in one of the poses used for meditation or pranayama. Inhale quietly through the nose and slowly contract and lift the muscles of the anus and perineum. Hold the breath for a while and exhale quietly whilst relaxing the bandha. Repeat calmly a few times. After practising for a while, try to hold the bandha a little longer while breathing normally.

Name

Uddiyana means to fly up, and *bandha* means to bind.

Effect

Uddiyana bandha is an important exercise. It strengthens the respiratory organs and the heart and makes them supple. It eradicates all nervous ailments in the area of the diaphragm, stomach and abdomen. It facilitates digestion and helps to get rid of accumulated poisonous material in the digestive tract. Uddiyana bandha is one of the best exercises for the abdominal organs. It strengthens the liver, spleen and bladder, removes stasis of blood and eases the pressure on the blood vessels. This bandha counteracts flabbiness in the abdomen, strengthens the genitals and facilitates the function of these organs. Thus the bandha may remove undesirable irritation of the genitals and control involuntary emissions in men, as well as relieving irregular and painful menses.

Uddiyana bandha is a great help in the transformation of sexual power to spiritual and mental energy. On the spiritual plane the posture, both as an independent exercise and in connection with pranayama, is used to assist the awakening of the Kundalini Shakti (see p. 157).

In general

Take care that the abdominal muscles are relaxed before the drawing up and in of the abdominal region, which is assisted by the expansion of the rib cage. Slightly raise the shoulders and tighten the neck a little, but avoid lowering the chest. Take the shoulders back a fraction and lean the whole upper part of the body slightly forwards. Relax all the muscles and lower the diaphragm before exhaling. Uddiyana is easiest to learn in a standing position, later one may do it sitting in padmasana (see p. 112). Be careful if you have a weak heart or chronic gastritis and enteritis. The exercise should not be done by women in the change of life or young girls before they are fully mature. It must not be done during or just after pregnancy or menstruation. It is important to do uddiyana on an empty stomach, or to wait for at least 3 hours after a meal. The exercise should not be done if pain is felt.

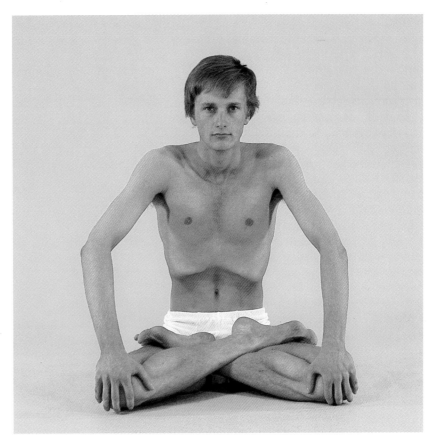

Duration

In the beginning, hold the bandha for a couple of seconds, and repeat 3-4 times. Slowly increase the time as long as you feel comfortable and increase the number of repetitions to 6 times.

Technique

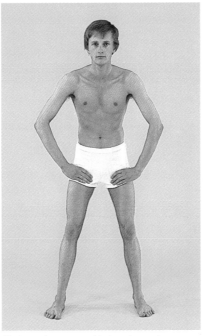

Sit in padmasana with hands on knees, or stand with legs apart, knees slightly bent and hands high up on the thighs, leaning the trunk forward slightly. Exhale forcibly, pulling the abdomen in and rounding the shoulders forward.

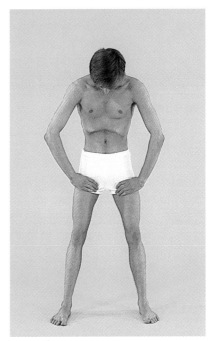

Bend chin to chest, relax the abdominal muscles while expanding the ribs, thereby lifting the diaphragm and creating a cavity under the ribs. Retain for as long as it is comfortable. Lift the head and inhale slowly, lowering the diaphragm.

Maha mudra

Name

Maha mudra means the great closing.

Effect

The practice of maha mudra brings about a moderate stretch of the complete back, stimulating the nerves and spreading a pleasant, relaxing warmth. It stimulates and facilitates blood circulation and may cure haemorrhoids, gastritis, bad digestion, enlarged spleen and diseases of the lungs. However, the most important thing about this mudra is its influence on the nervous system and the mind. With maha mudra you get a firm hold, so to speak, on all nervous restlessness in the body. It brings order and harmony to the nerve currents and creates a feeling of lightness and strength. At the same time it calms the emotions, automatic thought currents and irritation in the sense organs. It helps to collect the mind and is therefore well suited as a preliminary exercise before meditation and pranayama.

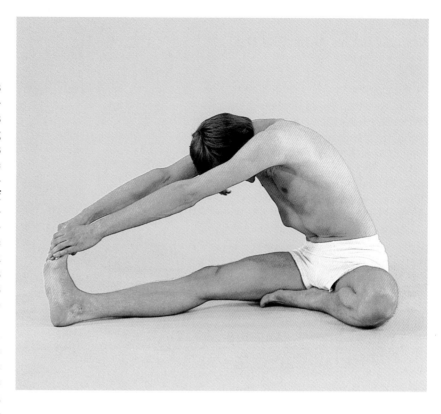

In general

In maha mudra you may either press the heel against the anus, or put the heel in towards the body, with the foot along the opposite thigh. Bend forward and grasp the foot, taking care to rest on both buttocks and not to lean to the sides. Try to keep the bent knee on the floor and the other leg straight. The effect is increased when you press the chin as far down toward the breast-bone as possible, and straighten up the back so that the neck and the area between the shoulder blades are stretched.

Should any tension arise from fixing the gaze between the eyebrows, concentrate on the point with eyes shut.

Duration

Keep the posture for as long as it feels pleasant to do so, with retained breath (antara kumbhaka). Repeat a couple of times to each side.

Technique

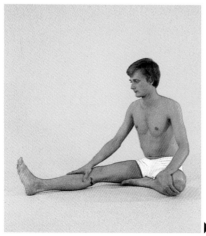

Sit on the left foot, with the heel pressing against the anus, and the right leg stretched forward, toes pointing up.

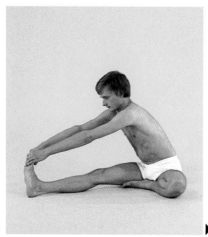

Grasp the toes of the right foot with both hands, keeping the back straight. Inhale slowly and hold the breath.

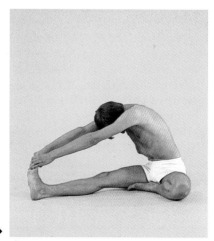

Apply jalandhara bandha (p. 120) and fix the gaze between the eyebrows. Hold the pose as long as it is comfortable. Raise the head and exhale slowly. Repeat on the left side.

Name

Maha bandha means the great lock.

Effect

This very effective bandha combines all the advantages of the jalandhara, mula and uddiyana bandhas. Further, exhalation in maha bandha has its own dynamics, which influences the nervous system directly, and purifies and activates the countless fine or subtle nerve currents which are otherwise inactive. These energies express themselves, not as muscular or other organic forces, but as a subtle energy field flowing through the physical as well as the mental plane. Maha bandha has a purifying and preventive effect. It counteracts degeneration, and facilitates meditation. Yogis use this bandha as a part of spiritual exercises to raise the Kundalini Shakti to higher planes.

In general

In order to obtain maximum benefit from this exercise, it is important that it is performed regularly over a long period. Unfortunately it may be difficult to learn it correctly on your own. Begin the exercise with a forceful and deep exhalation. Contract the anus and the perineum (mula bandha), and draw the abdomen in and up; then inhale through the nose by expanding the chest to the sides. This requires some practice, as you will be apt to gasp for air at the beginning, owing to the low pressure in the chest cavity. After exhaling, perform the chin lock (jalandhara bandha), and retain the posture for as long as it is comfortable. Complete the exercise by straightening up the head and calmly exhaling while the diaphragm and abdomen are lowered, and the mula bandha is relaxed. Should you experience any unpleasant pressures, pains or tension, then you are not doing the exercise correctly. In this case you should learn the technique from an experienced instructor.

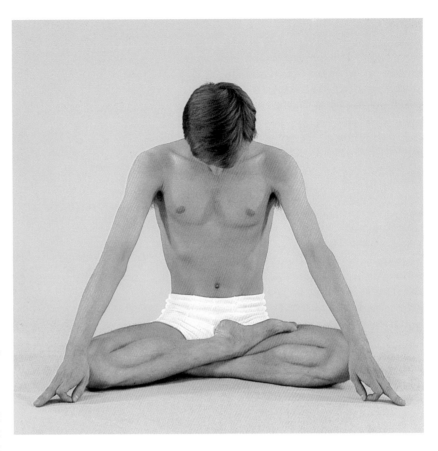

Duration

Maha bandha is usually performed once to each side, i.e. with different position of the legs, unless one is under the guidance of an experienced teacher and uses the exercise in connection with spiritual yoga training.

Technique

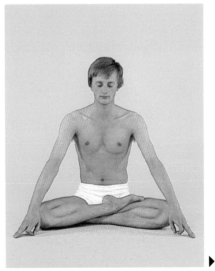

Sit erect with the left heel pressing against the anus. Place the right instep in the left groin and the hands on the knees. Exhale, apply mula bandha, and pull the abdomen well in and up (uddiyana bandha).

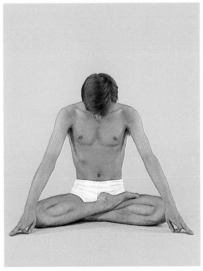

Inhale quietly, expanding the ribs. Hold the breath, performing jalandhara bandha (p. 120). Concentrate on the Kundalini (vital power) in the Sushumna (the spine). Relax the bandhas and exhale slowly. Repeat with the opposite leg position.

123

Maha veda

Name

Maha means great, and *veda* means penetration. The spiritual aim of this exercise is to make the Kundalini Shakti penetrate the sushumna nadi (an important nerve channel) in the spinal cord and rise up to the static centre of power in the crown of the head.

Effect

The full effect of maha veda is attained when it is done in connection with the two previous exercises, maha mudra and maha bandha. Maha veda further purifies the body and nerves, activates the latent energies and makes the body light. It helps digestion and respiration and counteracts disease and degeneration. When the exercise is combined with the other mudras and bandhas and is followed by pranayama and meditation in a regular daily programme, you gradually attain the threefold purity (in the body, nadis and mind), which is necessary in order to make the Kundalini Shakti rise to higher planes and thereby open the way to the highest state of consciousness.

In general

The posture must be firm, stable and immovable. Avoid sudden, jerky and restless movements when you raise and lower the body, as it will disturb

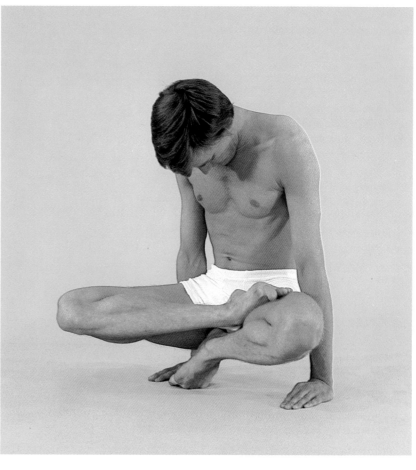

the calm flow of prana created by the posture. If you have weak wrists, you can clench your fists and rest on the knuckles. In that case it is best to use the leg posture where the heel is held against the anus during the whole exercise.

Duration

Keep the body lifted as long as it is comfortable to hold your breath. Maha veda may be done a couple of times in padmasana, or once on each heel, unless the exercise is a part of your spiritual training.

Technique

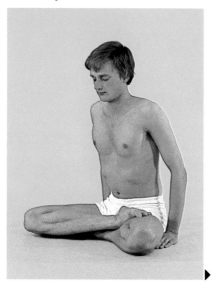

Sit erect with the left heel against the anus, the right foot by the left groin, and the palms on the floor by the buttocks. Inhale slowly.

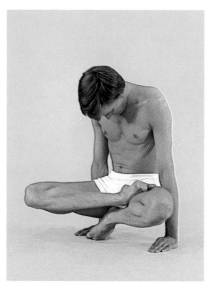

Perform jalandhara bandha (p. 120) and lift the buttocks off the floor. The pose should be firm. Lower the buttocks gently, lift the head and exhale.

Variation

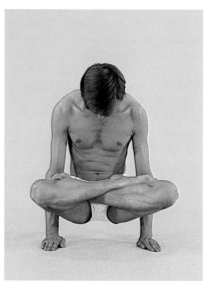

Maha veda may also be performed with the legs in padmasana (p. 112).

Chapter 4
Breathing exercises

The yoga breathing exercises consist of two main groups: the first comprising simple forms of deep regular breathing, and the other mainly very slow and deep breaths with kumbhaka (breath retention). The first group is done for the purpose of improving respiration and general health, often in connection with yoga asanas. The second group comprises the actual pranayama exercises which form a separate discipline and are normally done as part of a spiritual yoga training. In this chapter we describe a few important forms of breathing, which are easy to learn on your own, whereas the more advanced pranayama exercises require competent guidance.

Breathing exercises should be done in an undisturbed, clean and well-ventilated place. It is best to do the exercises on an empty stomach. Take care that the nostrils are clean, either by performing Jala Neti (p. 22), or by carefully sucking up a little tepid salt water into the nostrils and blowing it out through one nostril at a time. In both cases be careful to expel all the water.

The complete breath

Effect

The complete breath is the basis of respiration in almost all yoga exercises. This kind of breathing is necessary not only for the exercises to be performed correctly, but also in order to understand and be aware of the function of breathing itself.

In the complete breath you inhale 7-8 times more air than usual, and thereby attain the best possible ventilation of the lung tissue. This increases the removal of waste products and disease germs, especially in those areas of the lungs that are not active in normal breathing. Deep, calm breathing is thus very important for the health of the lungs and the purification and oxidation of the blood.

By regular and systematic practice of complete breathing, you experience and learn to understand the many almost imperceptible mechanisms of respiration. As a result of being able to breathe with minimum effort, you automatically relax those respiratory muscles that are not directly active while breathing. This also helps to lessen general tension in the organism.

When you consciously control the respiratory impulses in this way, with slow, deep and even breathing, the nerve energy (prana) begins to flow freely and unhindered through the whole organism, so that the body is felt as light and vital, while the mind becomes calm and balanced. You may thereby control emotions and gather the scattered thoughts. It is this function of breathing that gives an insight into the inner conscious life, from which you gain an idea of the real meaning of inner peace and quiet.

The complete breath exercises and strengthens the respiratory muscles. By relaxing the organism and bringing order into the rhythm of the individual, strain on the heart is relieved and blood circulation promoted. Breathing exercises are therefore effective in combating poor circulation, as well as ailments of the heart and blood vessels.

In general

The complete breath consists of three phases. The inhalation begins by lowering the diaphragm with breathing in

Technique

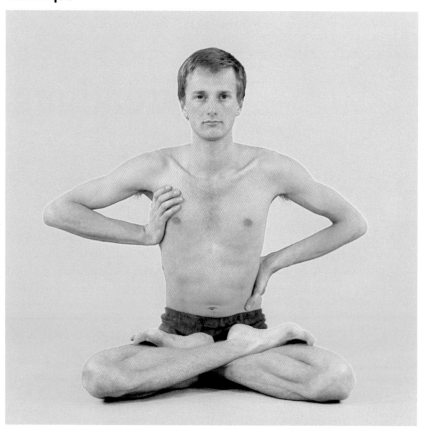

Sit relaxed, with a straight back. Place the left hand at the waist with the thumb forward and the other fingers back, and the right hand under the armpit with thumb behind. Relax the face, throat and jaws. Inhale quietly through the nose, feeling the current of air on the soft palate. Relax the abdomen and fill the lungs from the bottom upward, expanding the waist and loins. Continue the inhalation, gradually expanding the rib cage as the lungs are filled to the apex. Exhale gradually from the bottom of the lungs, contracting the abdomen and loins, and then slowly lowering the ribs. Exhale as much as possible without strain. The filling and emptying of the lungs should be done smoothly, with inhalations and exhalations of equal duration. This may also be practised lying on the back with the same hand position. When you are familiar with this, do the complete breath with the arms relaxed by the sides or as shown under meditation postures (pp. 111-112).

the lower part of the lungs. In the next phase the ribs are lifted, so that the chest is expanded, and lastly, the upper part of the lungs is activated. In the final phase of a deep inhalation the abdominal wall has a tendency to draw itself in a little. This entails an upward-directed pressure on the diaphragm, which helps to start the process of exhalation easily and smoothly. Exhalation should take place calmly and in a continuous movement that begins from the bottom of the lungs. When the ribs are lowered in the final stage of exhalation, the abdomen has an in-built tendency to expand and prepare for the next inhalation. When you begin to breathe deeply and be aware of the breath, the transition between exhalation and inhalation may often give

rise to small jerky tensions that move upward from the diaphragm and interrupt breathing. This may usually be overcome by a slight exaggeration of the muscle movements. During inhalation you may thus begin by pressing the stomach a little outwards and then let the ribs lift the chest as far upwards as possible, without tension. At the same time, mentally follow the inflow of air that fills the lungs from the floor to the apex. During exhalation you may likewise begin to draw in the stomach very slightly and then only let the ribs be lowered in a relaxed movement, while the air slowly flows out. This light stress in the lower respiratory muscles works as a bandha (bond) that absorbs any tension which may arise in the transitional phases of breathing.

By consciously working with the respiratory movements, the respiratory muscles become strong and relaxed, while breathing becomes deeper and easier. After some practice you learn to co-ordinate the muscle movements, so that all the breathing phases become smooth and continuous in one single flowing movement. When you feel the breath flowing freely, you may cease directing the muscle movements and instead concentrate on the smooth inflow and outflow of breath. This is done by adjusting the rate of breathing. In yoga breathing exercises it is essential to breathe as slowly as is possible without tensions, irregularities or other discomfort arising: if you breathe *too* slowly, tensions will arise which make the air-stream and muscle movements irregular. This may be overcome by breathing a little faster and concentrating on making the air-stream equal in the different phases of breathing. When you find your own personal rhythm, a deep harmony of the various energy impulses of the organism is attained. This may completely change the body concept, allowing breathing to be experienced as a free and unhindered flow of vitality, with a feeling of lightness.

The complete breath may be performed in most situations – sitting, lying, standing or walking. You may do this breathing before, during and after physical exercise, during rest, mental exertion and after a meal, and so on. There are no limitations attached to deep breathing, but you should ensure that it is not obstructed by tight clothing or forward-bending postures.

If you experience difficulty in doing the complete breath, it may help to practise the abdominal, rib and collar-bone breathing separately. When these three phases are combined in a single breathing, it is called the complete breath. These three partial kinds of breathing may be learnt either sitting or lying, and by using the hands you can easily perceive the muscle and lung movements of each phase. In practising you should separate each breathing phase as far as possible, and repeat each one only 5-10 times.

Variation

When you have become quite familiar with the complete breath, you may reinforce its balancing effect by imagining that the current of inhaled air passes only through the left nostril and that exhalation takes place through the right, and that the next inhalation takes place through the right nostril followed by exhalation through the left. By imagining this alternating stream in the nostrils you strengthen your power of concentration and create a harmonious balance of the nerve currents (prana). You should not try to distend or contract the nostrils, only follow the changing currents mentally. Ensure that the eyes do not follow the movement but remain relaxed and closed. After some practice you can actually feel how your concentrated imagination can influence the air current in the nostrils. This kind of breathing is called *triangular breathing*.

Preliminary exercises

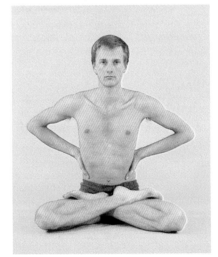

Abdominal breathing can be practised with hands on the waist, thumbs pointing forward and the other fingers behind. Inhale quietly through the nose. The abdominal muscles should be relaxed, allowing the free movement of the diaphragm to expand the bottom of the lungs. Feel the loins lifting on inhalation, but avoid lifting the ribs. Exhale quietly, feeling the contraction of the loins and waist. In a sitting position, the abdominal muscles contract in deep exhalations, but should relax prior to inhalation.

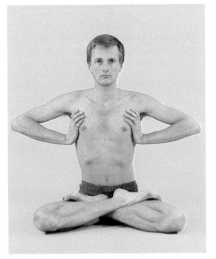

Costal breathing can be practised with the hands as high under the armpits as possible, the thumbs pointing backward and the other fingers forward. Inhale quietly and fill the middle part of the lungs without expanding the abdomen or loins. Feel the ribs lifting outward and upward. Exhale in a relaxed way and feel the ribs lowering again. You may isolate the costal breath by contracting the abdomen, but be sure to avoid tension in the shoulders or throat.

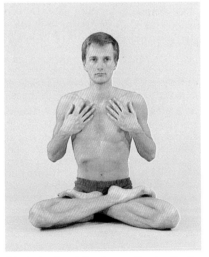

Clavicular breathing is practised with the palms high on the chest, fingers on the collar bone. Keep the abdomen slightly drawn in and try to avoid lifting the ribs. Inhale through the nose with small inhalations, filling the apex of the lungs little by little. Feel the breast-bone lifting. Some of the neck muscles are used in this kind of breathing. Exhale passively, quietly lowering the breast-bone. These three kinds of breathing are combined into one relaxed smooth movement in the complete breath.

Wave breathing

Effect

This kind of breathing is a variation of the complete breath which greatly strengthens the lung tissue and respiratory muscles, especially the diaphragm and the abdominal muscles. "Wave breathing" is an effective exercise to alleviate uncontrolled nervous activity in the solar plexus, constipation, air in the intestines, poor circulation, etc. This exercise counteracts involuntary emission of sperm. If you do it in bed early in the morning before rising, it activates blood circulation and nerve currents, eliminating sleepiness and lethargy. If this kind of breathing is done regularly every day, it will be a great help in retaining good health.

In general

Wave breathing is usually done lying on the back with an empty stomach. The pulling up must be done in one smooth and calm movement, and not be exaggerated or give rise to any pain. Drawing up an distension must take place in a continuous rhythm whilst the breath is held. Find a number of movements suitable for your constitution. The exercise must not cause any strain or leave you short of breath. Use the necessary muscles only, and avoid tension in the body, especially in the face and shoulders.

Technique

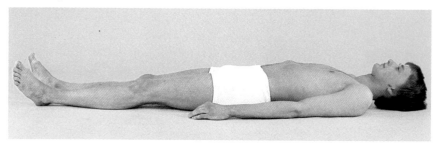

Lie on the back, elongate and relax the spine. Those with excessive spinal curvature can bend the knees and place the soles of the feet on the floor. Inhale moderately through the nose.

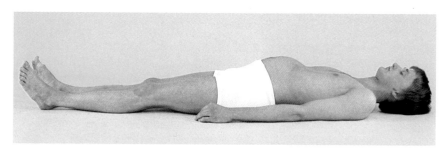

Hold the breath. Push the diaphragm downward, thereby lifting the abdominal wall. Avoid moving the back, so that it can remain relaxed and flat on the floor during the whole exercise.

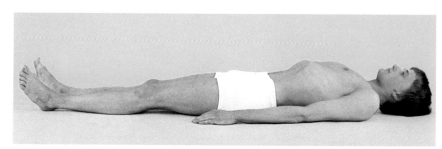

Pull the diaphragm upward, thereby lowering the abdominal wall and expanding the rib cage. This down–up movement may be repeated a few times according to capacity.

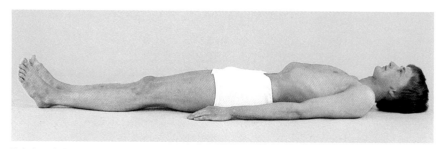

Exhale quietly. Remain with lungs emptied of air. Lift up the diaphragm, expanding the rib cage, so that the abdominal wall forms a cavity.

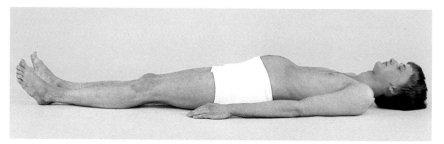

Push the diaphragm down, raising the abdominal wall. The up-down movement may be repeated a few times. Relax and inhale. Beginners may repeat this cycle a few times, gradually increasing the number of wave movements according to capacity. Advanced yoga students may perform up to 5 rounds consisting of 5-10 wave movements.

Effect

This yogic breathing exercise is primarily intended to regulate and balance the nervous impulses and prana currents which form the basis of respiration, and to purify the subtle nerve channels, thus vitalising the organism. This exercise creates calmness and balance in the nervous system, purifies the thoughts, increases the power of concentration and eliminates agitation and painful emotions. It purifies the lungs and blood, normalises all the functions of the body and improves your state of health.

In general

Pranayama No. 1 must be done in a sitting posture and with a straight back. It is an advantage if you can do the exercise in padmasana (p. 112) or another meditation posture, but you may also sit in a chair, provided your back is relaxed and straight. Wait a couple of hours after a meal before doing the exercise. Pranayama should be a part of your daily programme after yoga postures. However, women should avoid doing pranayama during menstruation and pregnancy.

Pranayama No. 1 is a variation of the complete breath (p. 126). Begin by inhaling through the left nostril while you close the right nostril with the right thumb. At the end of the inhalation the left nostril is closed with the right ring and little fingers, and you exhale through the right nostril. Then inhale again through the right nostril and exhale through the left, while the right nostril is closed with the thumb. This is one round. You can do up to five rounds. Use the right hand to regulate the changing stream through the nostrils and do not lower the hand during the exercise. In the classical hand posture the arm is held close to the body, the thumb and the ring and the little fingers are kept straight, while the forefinger and second finger are bent down on the palm. If this posture is inconvenient, keep the arm in a horizontal position away from the body and, if you wish, use the thumb and forefinger on the nostrils. It is important to use a hand posture that does not give rise to any tension in the hand or tiredness in the arm. The hand and arm should not be moved more than necessary during the exercise, and it is important that the hand does not cover the active nostril, so that the air currents can pass freely. The posture must be comfortable, fixed and immovable, so that you can concentrate on the exercise undisturbed. When you have become accustomed to this pranayama, you can allow the inhalation and exhalation to take care of themselves. During inhalation imagine you are filled with health, strength, purity and all other good qualities you wish to acquire. During exhalation you may imagine that you are expelling disease, pain, degeneration and all the negative qualities of which you wish to be rid. These auto-suggestions must be performed systematically and with complete concentration, so that the desired results will come about.

Technique

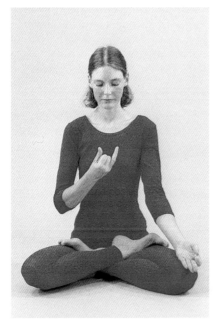 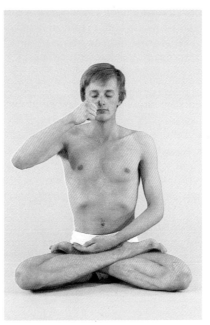 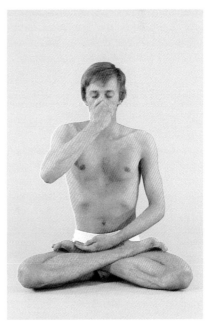

In the classical hand position the right hand is used to regulate the current of air through the nostrils. The thumb, ring and little fingers are stretched, whilst the index and middle fingers are bent toward the palm, with the arm resting lightly on the chest without hampering the expansion of the lungs.

If this arm position is unpleasant or hampers respiration, hold the arm away from the body, using the same position of the fingers, or you may close the right nostril with the thumb, and the left nostril with the index finger.

Close the right nostril with the right thumb, then inhale slowly and quietly through the left nostril. Then close the left nostril with the ring and little fingers, and exhale quietly through the right nostril. Again, inhale through the right nostril and exhale through the left one. This forms one round, repeat 2-5 times.

Chapter 5
Concentration exercises

The mind is a subtle force upheld by Consciousness. It has no form or colour of its own, but takes the form and colour of the thought object. The mind cannot live for a single second without thinking of something. Different thought forms arise incessantly on the conscious plane of the mind as waves on the surface of the sea. The more desires and thoughts that arise in the mind, the more restless and dissipated it becomes, and the more disturbed, tense and weary our condition. To empty the mind of desires and thoughts requires a serious effort in the form of a well-regulated life and systematic concentration exercises.

In yoga two forms of concentration are recognised: automatic concentration and concentration at will. Automatic concentration is developed in all life forms and is usually directed towards sense objects and pleasures; whereas concentration at will is developed only in human beings who deliberately practise concentration exercises.

Automatic concentration arises in the mind whether one wants it or not, and in the case of concentration on negative emotions, it may be positively harmful. Concentration at will, on the other hand, is always a voluntary process enabling withdrawal of the mind from a harmful, painful or undesirable state, and fixing it on something positive, strength-giving and elevating. Concentration of the mind at will helps to keep the mind calm and balanced, thus ensuring a state of permanent contentment, equilibrium and happiness.

Concentration of the mind at will is the essence of all yoga and meditation. Without concentration of the mind there can be no inner peace. If we are not able to practise this, we become helpless victims of the vicissitudes of life, whereas the power of concentration enables us to be masters of ourselves and of the vast inner world that in reality is as infinite as the outer universe.

Concentration exercises

Trataka

Trataka is an eye exercise that strengthens the eyesight (see p. 28) as well as improving the mental power of concentration. When doing trataka as a concentration exercise, you also fix the sight on an object or a single point; but apart from this you also try to concentrate your whole attention on this object, thereby excluding all other thoughts. In the beginning it is common for the eyes to water; this may be alleviated by blinking a couple of times. If you continue practising, you will be able to carry on for a longer time without blinking. Many find that their vision of the object of concentration wavers, or that it appears to grow bigger or smaller, so that concentration becomes difficult. These phenomena are quite normal and disappear after some practice. In the beginning it is not possible to focus your whole attention on the object of concentration, and you will experience a lot of distracting thoughts that arise unnoticed and often make you lose your absorption. When you again focus your concentration on the point, you should not become irritated owing to these repeated interruptions, or lose hope of being able to attain your goal. The ordinary untrained mind constantly changes form, and is prone to wander according to its whims and fancies. If the mind is very fickle, it may be a help to evolve a chain of thought concerning the object of concentration, while gazing at and observing it carefully. Now and then, you can also close your eyes and try to picture the object for as long as possible. After practising for some days, you will notice a distinct improvement in concentration and eyesight, and thoughts will be calmer.

The object of concentration should be simple and attractive. It may be a beautiful flower or a picture. A still candle flame in front of a dark background is very suitable, but a dark dot on a light background can also be used.

With practice, you will be able to fix your concentration on the object, and enjoy the resulting mental tranquillity. The sharpened power of concentration makes the thoughts clear and

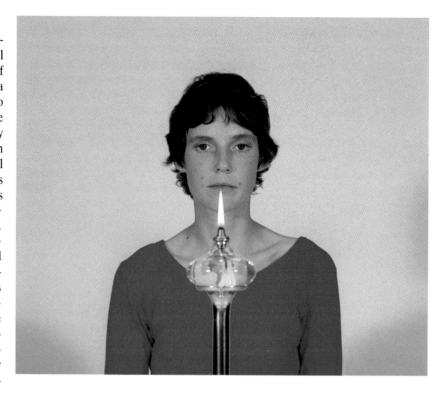

alert, and your conception of complex matters is enhanced. If you are able to concentrate deeply on the same object for a longer time, you will find that other sense impressions disappear completely. Complete silence prevails, and you will not even be aware that you are seated. If this state of concentration continues, the mind gradually severs contact with the sense of sight, and continues in the brain with the mental impression, quite independently of the external object. This is a very blissful state, where all the forces of the mind are united in the object, which will have a tendency to contract itself into a focal point. If concentration is continued, the idea of the body itself will disappear and respiration will almost be arrested. After some time even the point will merge into an all-pervading silvery light, which is finally merged in Infinity, where there is neither lightness nor darkness, neither time nor space. The process that enables the mind to concentrate fully on a single object for some seconds, is called *pratyahara*, and it signifies the first step in meditative concentration. When you become established in pra-

tyahara, you can withdraw the mind at will from the senses and fix it on a mental image under all conditions. A person who is able to do this has acquired a high degree of self mastery and enjoys deep peace and bliss.

Concentration on sound

Concentration on sound is another suitable exercise. To be used as an object of concentration, the sound must be soft and pleasant, and be either continuous or rhytmically repeated, such as the tick-tock of a clock. Irregular and varied musical sounds cannot be used for this purpose. In most cases a clock will be the best object of concentration. Sit still with straight back and closed eyes. Concentrate fully on the ticking sound. Let the mind become one with this sound and avoid all other disturbing thoughts.

When you have practised concentration and meditation for some time and the body and subtle yoga nadis (nerves) are purified, you may hear various mental sounds such as delicate, fine glass bells, distant stringed instruments or flute-like sounds. The last sound one hears is OM. This is

132

the Primal Sound, or the sound of the creative energy. It is different from all other sounds, and may only roughly be described as the sound of a distant waterfall, the continuous roar of the ocean, or the constant humming of a swarm of bees. The sound OM may be heard mentally when the Kundalini Shakti rises fully to the heart centre (Anahata Chakra), and it requires very hard work with meditation and mind-control to come to this point. For beginners it may be of considerable help to imagine the OM sound during the concentration exercises, and to concentrate on this allpervading cosmic sound. If you wish to read a detailed description of this subject: you will find it in *The Primal Power in Man* by Swami Narayanananda (published by N. U. Yoga Ashrama, Gylling, 8300 Odder, Denmark.

Concentration on void

Sit in a firm and comfortable posture with a straight back. Try not to think of anything at all. Empty the mind of all desires and thoughts. Forget the body and the senses, forget your worries and plans. Let all thoughts subside into the great silent void which is the original state of the mind, undisturbed by our incessant desires and thoughts. If you are able to empty the mind for just one moment, you will get a glimpse of Infinity or the Self, and you will have an idea of your own hidden powers and possibilities.

We experience this state of void in deep, dreamless sleep, and this is why we feel refreshed and rejuvenated after such a sleep. If you are able to empty the mind of desires and thoughts in the waking state, you will instantly be filled with strength and energy.

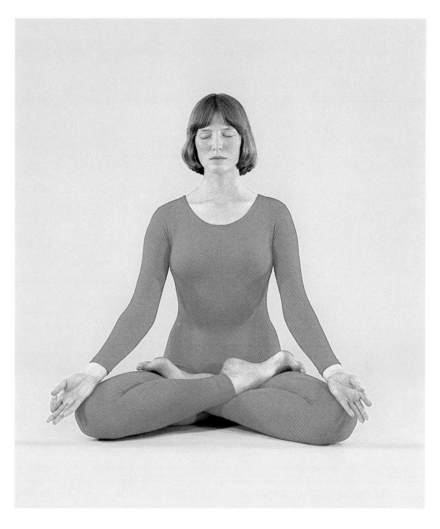

To concentrate the mind on void is a difficult art and requires practice over a long period. Even if you do not succeed at the beginning, the exercise in itself will give you peace and strength. As a concentration exercise consists in removing all mental images, no special method can be described, and each one has to find a way of emptying the mind of its objects. If you are able to continue this concentration without interruption for about half an hour, you may transcend the limits of the individual consciousness and merge in Cosmic Consciousness or Self-Realisation.

Chapter 6
Exercise series

In the following diagrams, 9 different series of yoga postures are proposed for your daily training programme. This series gives some examples of how a succession of yoga-asanas can be put together for individual needs.

If you have practised yoga postures for some time, you can learn to perceive the special effects arising from a combination of different exercises, and you can then devise your own programme. In most cases, exercise series No. 5 will be the best foundation for a continuing daily schedule, and if preferred, they can be combined with the different special exercises.

Exercise series No. 1   Beginners

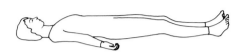

Savasana (p. 108) and
the complete breath (p. 126), 2 min.

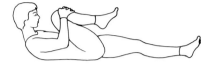

Dynamic pavanamuktasana (p. 82),
2-3 times.

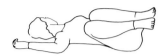

Back exercises No. 2, phases 2, 3, 4
(p. 35), 2-3 times.

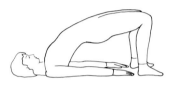

Kandhara preliminary exercise No. 1
(p. 80), twice.

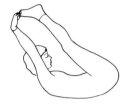

Halasana preliminary exercise No. 1
(p. 59), twice.

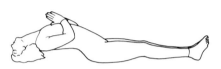

Matsyasana preliminary exercise No. 1
(p. 61), ½ min.

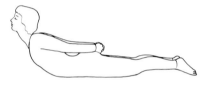

Bhujangasana preliminary exercise No. 1
(p. 63), twice.

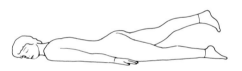

Salabhasana preliminary exercise No. 1
(p. 65), twice with each leg.

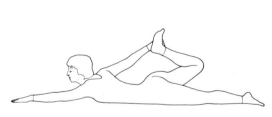

Dhanurasana preliminary exercise No. 2
(p. 67), once or twice to each side.

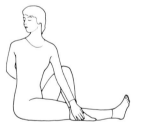

Ardha matsyendrasana preliminary exercise
No. 2 (p. 69), once or twice to each side.

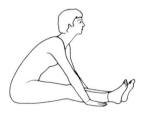

Paschimottanasana preliminary exercise
No. 2, (p. 71), ½-1 min.

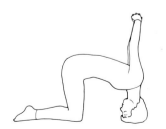

Sirshasana preliminary exercise No. 1
(p. 53), ½ min.

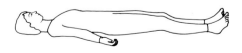

The complete breath (p. 126), 2 min.
Savasana (p. 108), 10 min.

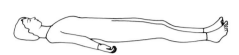

The complete breath (p. 126), 1 min.

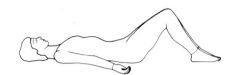

Wave breathing (p. 128), 3 times.

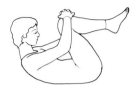

Back exercise No. 2 (p. 35), once.

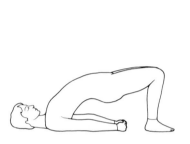

Kandhara preliminary exercise No. 2 (p. 80), once.

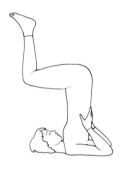

Sarvangasana preliminary exercise No. 1 (p. 56), ½ min.

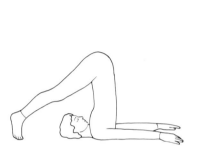

Halasana (p. 58), ½ min.

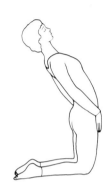

Ustrasana preliminary exercise No. 2 (p. 93), 3 times.

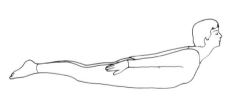

Bhujangasana preliminary exercise No. 2 (p. 63), twice.

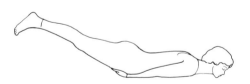

Salabhasana preliminary exercise No. 2 (p. 65), twice.

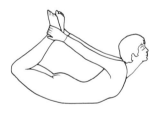

Dhanurasana preliminary exercise No. 5, once or twice.

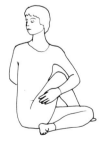

Ardha matsyendrasana preliminary exercise No. 6 (p. 69), ½ min. to each side.

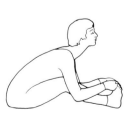

Paschimottanasana preliminary exercise No. 3 (p. 71), twice.

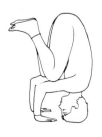

Sirshasana preliminary exercise No. 3 (p. 53), ½-1 min.

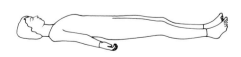

The complete breath, variation (p. 127), 2 min. Savasana (p. 108), 10 min.

Exercise series No. 3   For trained students with back problems

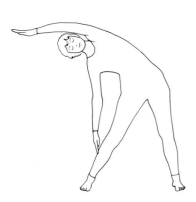

Trikonasana (p. 104), 3 times to each side.

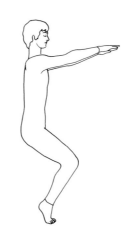

Utkatasana (p. 106), 3 times.

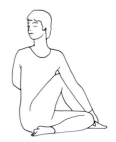

Ardha matsyendrasana (p. 68), 2 min.

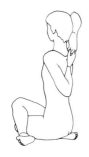

Gomukhasana (p. 84), 1-2 min. to each side.

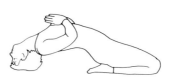

Supta vajrasana (p. 74), 2 min.

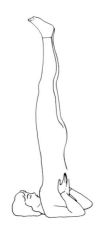

Sarvangasana (p. 54), 3 min.

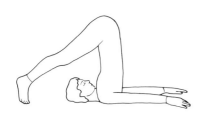

Halasana (p. 58), 3 min.

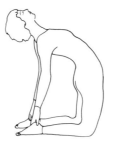

Ustrasana (p. 92), 1-2 min.

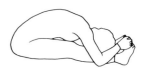

Paschimottanasana (p. 70), 2 min.

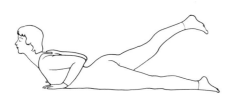

Bhujangasana, variation No. 2 (p. 63), with each leg and with both legs.

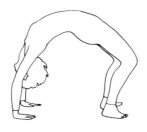

Chakrasana (p. 78), 1-2 min.

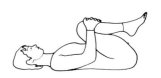

Pavanamuktasana (p. 82), 3 min.
Savasana (p. 108), 10 min.

Exercise series No. 4   For trained students, to strengthen concentration

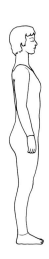

Stand with straight back, close your eyes, and watch your breathing, 1 min.

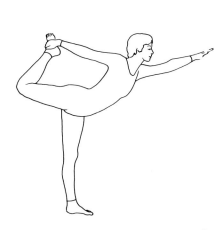

Natarajasana (p. 102), ½-1 min. to each side.

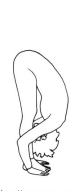

Paschimottanasana, variation No. 6 (p. 71), ½-1 min.

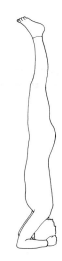

Sirshasana (p. 49), 2 min.

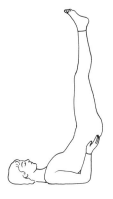

Viparita karani (p. 57), 5 min.

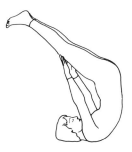

Sarvangasana preliminary exercise No. 3 (p. 56), 2 min.

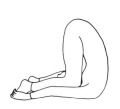

Halasana, variation No. 3 (p. 59), 3 min.

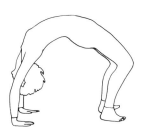

Chakrasana (p. 78), ½-1 min.

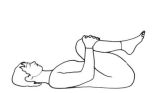

Pavanamuktasana, (p. 82), 2 min.

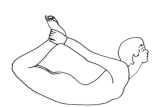

Dhanurasana (p. 66), twice.

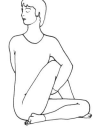

Ardha matsyendrasana variation No. 1 (p. 69), 2 min.

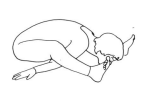

Kurmasana (p. 81), 1-1½ min.

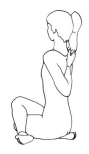

Gomukhasana (p. 84), 1 min. to each side.

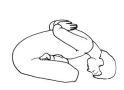

Yoga mudra (p. 114), 1-2 min.

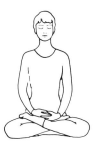

Padmasana (p. 112), the complete breath, variation (p. 127), 5 rounds.

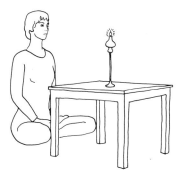

Trataka (pp. 28 and 132), 1-2 min.

Exercise series No. 5   For trained students, suitable for spiritual training

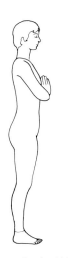

Suryanamaskar (p. 116-117), twice.

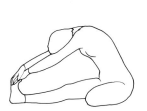

Maha mudra (p. 122), twice to each side.

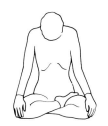

Maha bandha (p. 123), twice to each side.

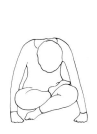

Maha veda (p. 124), twice.

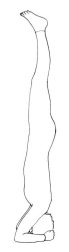

Sirshasana (p. 49), 2 min.

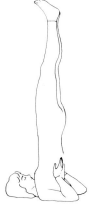

Sarvangasana (p. 54), 3 min.

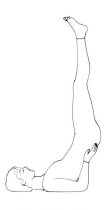

Viparita karani (p. 57), 5 min.

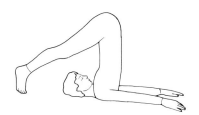

Halasana (p. 58), 3 min.

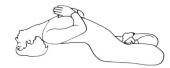

Matsyasana (p. 60), 2 min.

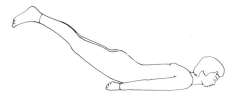

Salabhasana (p. 64), 4 times.

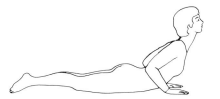

Bhujangasana (p. 62), 4 times.

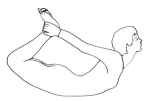

Dhanurasana (p. 66), 1-2 min.

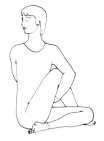

Ardha matsyendrasana (p. 68), 2 min.

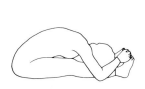

Paschimottanasana (p. 70), 1½-2 min.

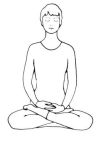

The complete breath, variation (p. 127), 5 times.

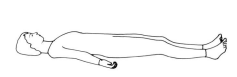

Savasana (p. 108), 10 min.

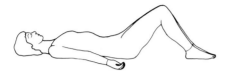

The complete breath (p. 126), and
wave breathing (p. 128), 3 times.

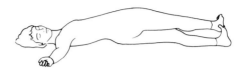

Back exercise No. 3 (p. 36), phases 1-6 and 8.

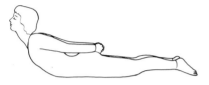

Bhujangasana preliminary exercise No. 1
(p. 63), twice.

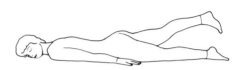

Salabhasana preliminary exercise No. 1
(p. 65), 3 times with each leg.

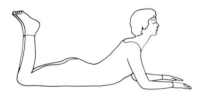

Dhanurasana preliminary exercise No. 3
(p. 67), twice.

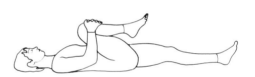

Pavanamuktasana (p. 82), 3 min.

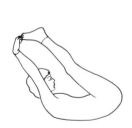

Halasana preliminary exercise No. 1
(p. 59), ½-1 min.

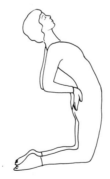

Ustrasana preliminary exercise
No. 1 (p. 93), ½ min.

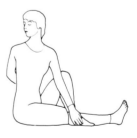

Ardha matsyendrasana preliminary exercise
No. 1 (p. 69), twice to each side.

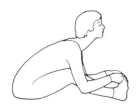

Paschimottanasana preliminary
exercise No. 3 (p. 71), ½-1 min.

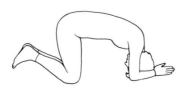

Sirshasana preliminary exercise No. 2
(p. 53), 1 min.

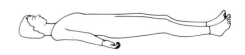

The complete breath, variation (p. 127),
5 times and Savasana (p. 108), 10 min.

Exercise series No. 7 For the elderly

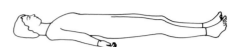

The complete breath (p. 126), 2 min.

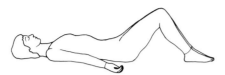

Wave breathing (p. 128), 3 times.

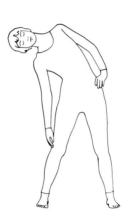

Trikonasana preliminary exercise No. 1 (p. 105), 3 times to each side.

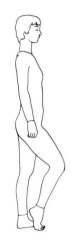

Leg and foot exercise No. 12 (p. 45), the whole series.

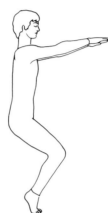

Utkatasana (p. 106), 2-3 times.

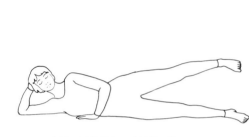

Leg and foot exercise No. 7 (p. 42), once to each side.

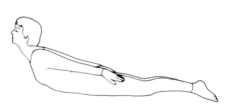

Bhujangasana preliminary exercise No. 2 (p. 63), twice.

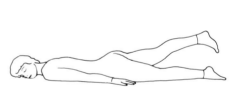

Salabhasana preliminary exercise No. 1 (p. 65), twice with each leg.

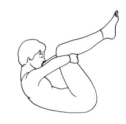

Halasana preliminary exercise No. 2 (p. 58), 1-2 min.

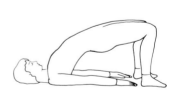

Kandharasana preliminary exercise No. 1 (p. 80), twice.

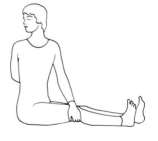

Ardha matsyendrasana preliminary exercise No. 1 (p. 69), twice to each side.

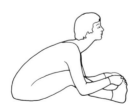

Paschimottanasana preliminary exercise No. 3 (p. 71), twice.

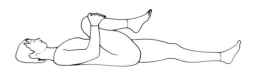

Pavanamuktasana (p. 82), 3 min.

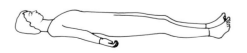

The complete breath, variation (p. 127), and Savasana (p. 108), 10 min.

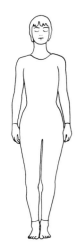

The complete breath (p. 126), 1-2 min. (sitting in a chair).

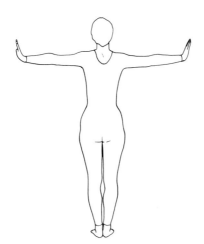

Shoulder exercise No. 4, (p. 31), 3 times (sitting, if you like).

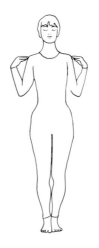

Shoulder exercise No. 7 (p. 32), 3 times (sitting if you like).

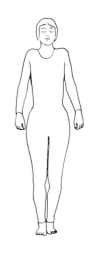

Shoulder exercise No. 9 (p. 32), twice (sitting, if you like).

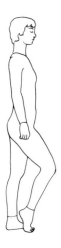

Leg and foot exercise No. 12 (p. 45).

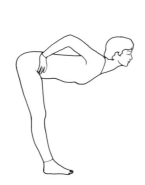

Ardha chandrasana, preliminary exercise (p. 99), twice.

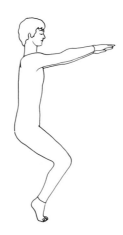

Utkatasana (p. 106), 2-3 times.

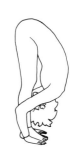

Paschimottanasana, variation No. 6 (p. 71), twice.

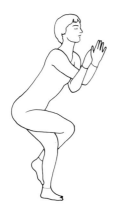

Garudasana (p. 100), ½ min. on each side.

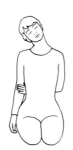

Neck exercixe No. 1 (p. 26), twice.

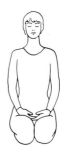

The complete breath, variation (p. 126), 5 rounds (sitting relaxed with eyes shut).

Exercise series No. 9 To relieve stress

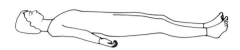

The complete breath (p. 126), 2 min.

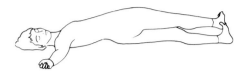

Back exercise No. 3 (p. 36), whole series.

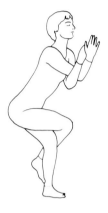

Garudasana (p. 100),
1 min. on each side.

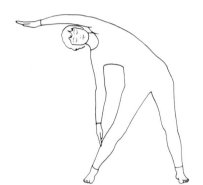

Trikonasana (p. 104),
twice on each side.

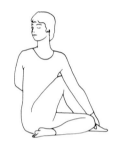

Ardha matsyendrasana
(p. 68), 1-2 min.

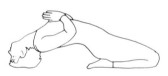

Supta vajrasana (p. 74), 1-2 min.

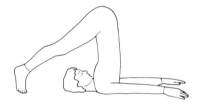

Halasana (p. 58), 2 min.

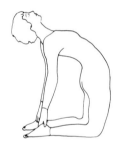

Ustrasana (p. 92), ½-1 min.

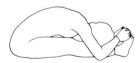

Paschimottanasana (p. 70), 1-2 min.

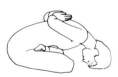

Yoga mudra (p. 114), 2 min.

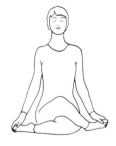

Samkatasana (p. 98), 1 min.

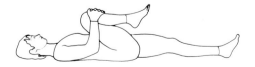

Pavanamuktasana (p. 82), 3 min.

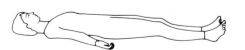

The complete breath, variation (p. 127),
5 times. Savasana (p. 108), 15 min.

Supplement
Anatomical atlas

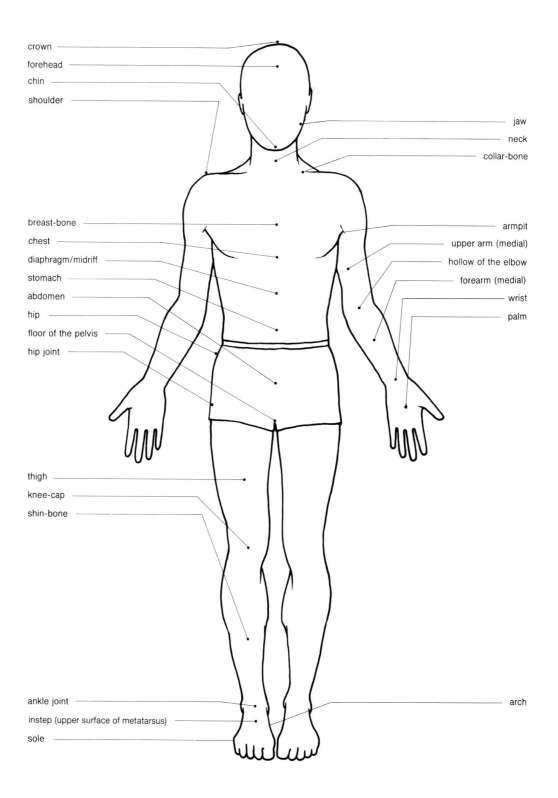

crown

forehead

chin

shoulder

jaw

neck

collar-bone

breast-bone

chest

diaphragm/midriff

stomach

abdomen

hip

floor of the pelvis

hip joint

armpit

upper arm (medial)

hollow of the elbow

forearm (medial)

wrist

palm

thigh

knee-cap

shin-bone

ankle joint

arch

instep (upper surface of metatarsus)

sole

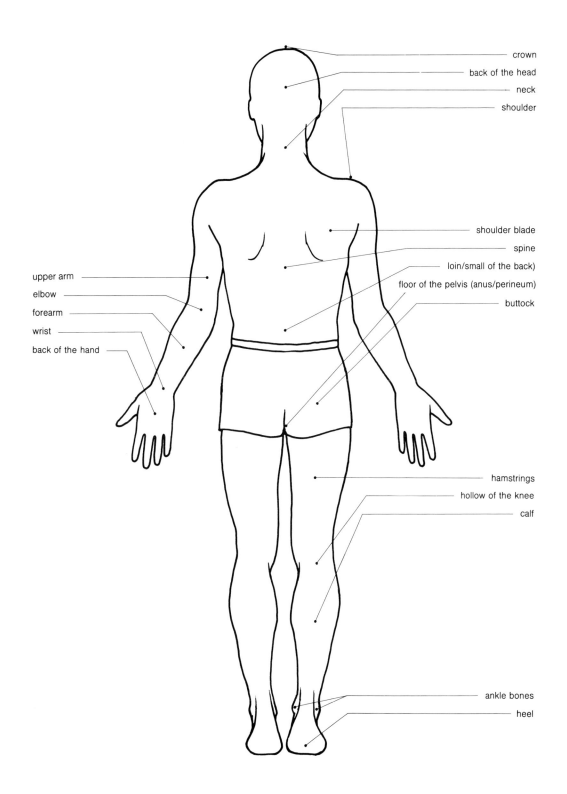

crown

back of the head

neck

shoulder

shoulder blade

spine

loin/small of the back)

floor of the pelvis (anus/perineum)

buttock

upper arm

elbow

forearm

wrist

back of the hand

hamstrings

hollow of the knee

calf

ankle bones

heel

The muscular system (posterior)

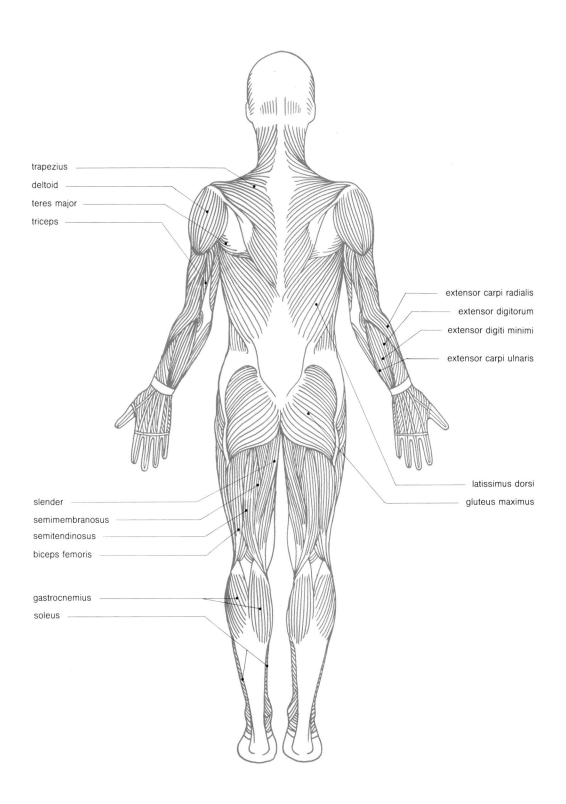

trapezius

deltoid

teres major

triceps

extensor carpi radialis

extensor digitorum

extensor digiti minimi

extensor carpi ulnaris

latissimus dorsi

gluteus maximus

slender

semimembranosus

semitendinosus

biceps femoris

gastrocnemius

soleus

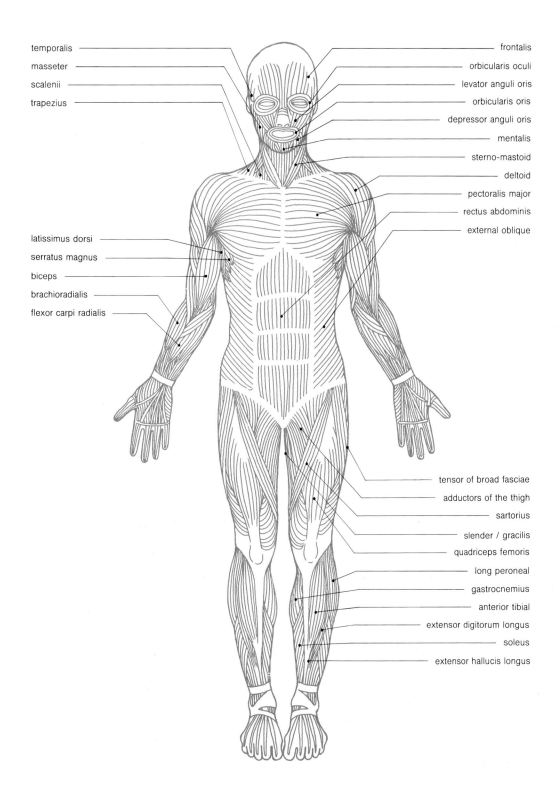

temporalis

masseter

scalenii

trapezius

frontalis

orbicularis oculi

levator anguli oris

orbicularis oris

depressor anguli oris

mentalis

sterno-mastoid

deltoid

pectoralis major

rectus abdominis

external oblique

latissimus dorsi

serratus magnus

biceps

brachioradialis

flexor carpi radialis

tensor of broad fasciae

adductors of the thigh

sartorius

slender / gracilis

quadriceps femoris

long peroneal

gastrocnemius

anterior tibial

extensor digitorum longus

soleus

extensor hallucis longus

The skeletal system

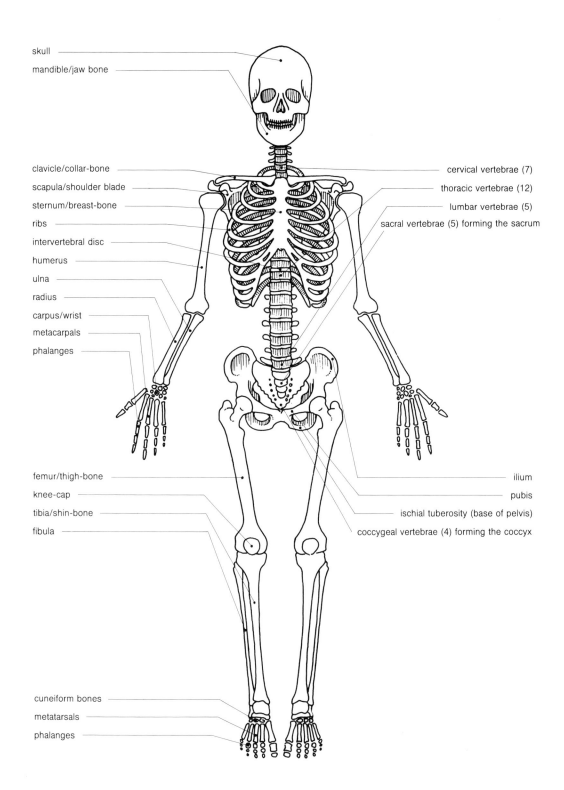

skull

mandible/jaw bone

clavicle/collar-bone

scapula/shoulder blade

sternum/breast-bone

ribs

intervertebral disc

humerus

ulna

radius

carpus/wrist

metacarpals

phalanges

cervical vertebrae (7)

thoracic vertebrae (12)

lumbar vertebrae (5)

sacral vertebrae (5) forming the sacrum

femur/thigh-bone

knee-cap

tibia/shin-bone

fibula

ilium

pubis

ischial tuberosity (base of pelvis)

coccygeal vertebrae (4) forming the coccyx

cuneiform bones

metatarsals

phalanges

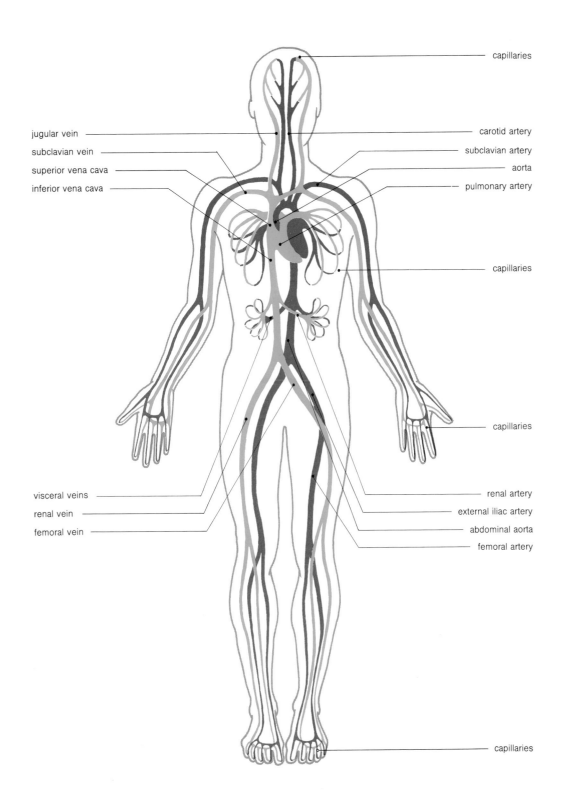

jugular vein

subclavian vein

superior vena cava

inferior vena cava

capillaries

carotid artery

subclavian artery

aorta

pulmonary artery

capillaries

capillaries

visceral veins

renal vein

femoral vein

renal artery

external iliac artery

abdominal aorta

femoral artery

capillaries

The digestive system

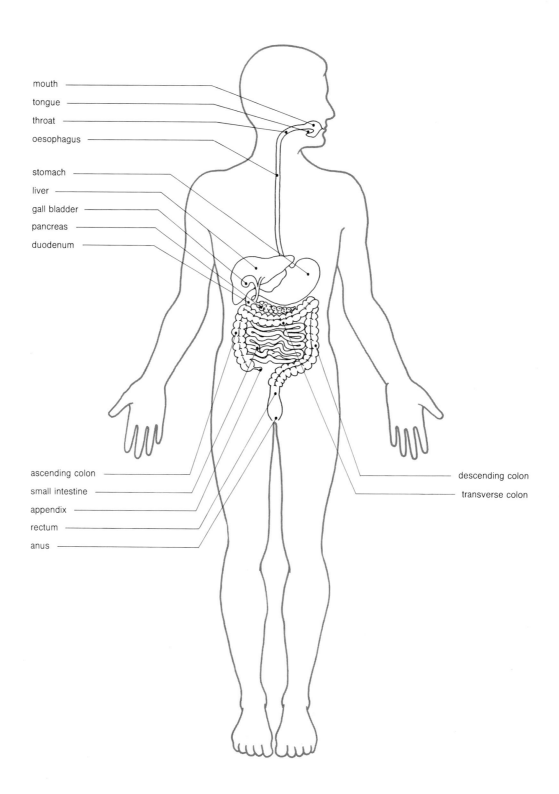

mouth

tongue

throat

oesophagus

stomach

liver

gall bladder

pancreas

duodenum

ascending colon

small intestine

appendix

rectum

anus

descending colon

transverse colon

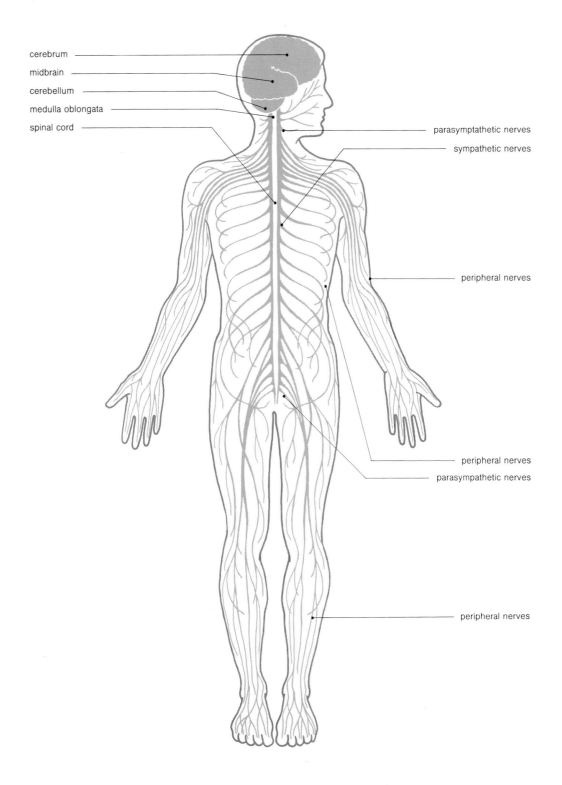

cerebrum
midbrain
cerebellum
medulla oblongata
spinal cord

parasymptathetic nerves
sympathetic nerves

peripheral nerves

peripheral nerves
parasympathetic nerves

peripheral nerves

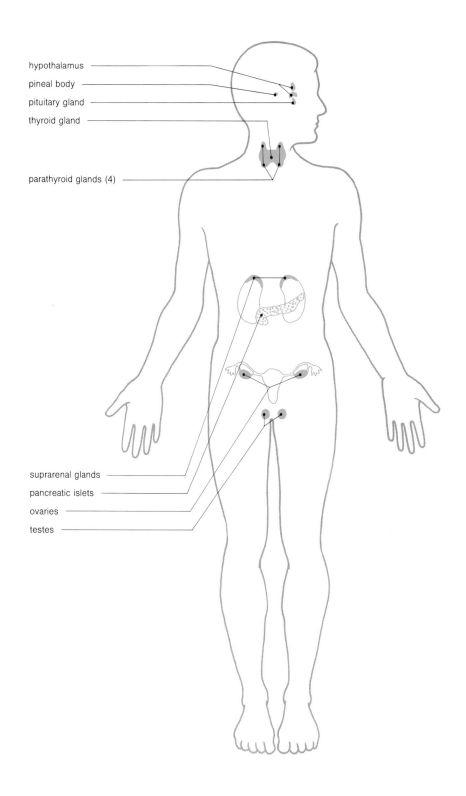

hypothalamus

pineal body

pituitary gland

thyroid gland

parathyroid glands (4)

suprarenal glands

pancreatic islets

ovaries

testes

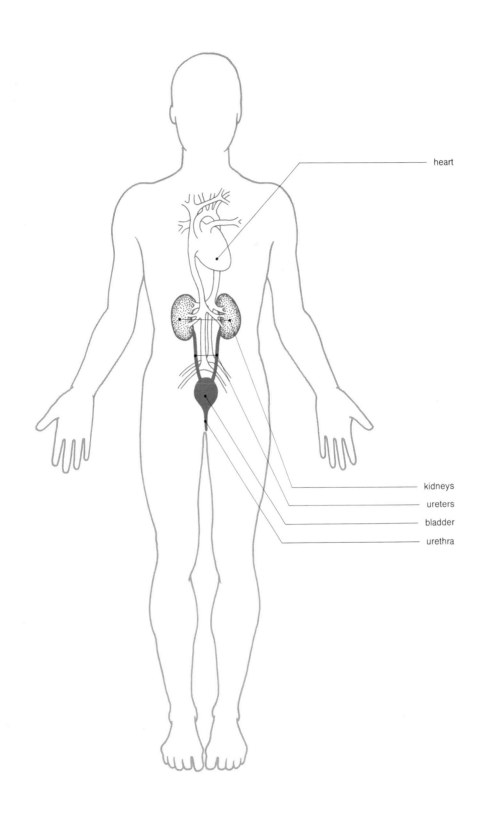

heart

kidneys

ureters

bladder

urethra

The respiratory system

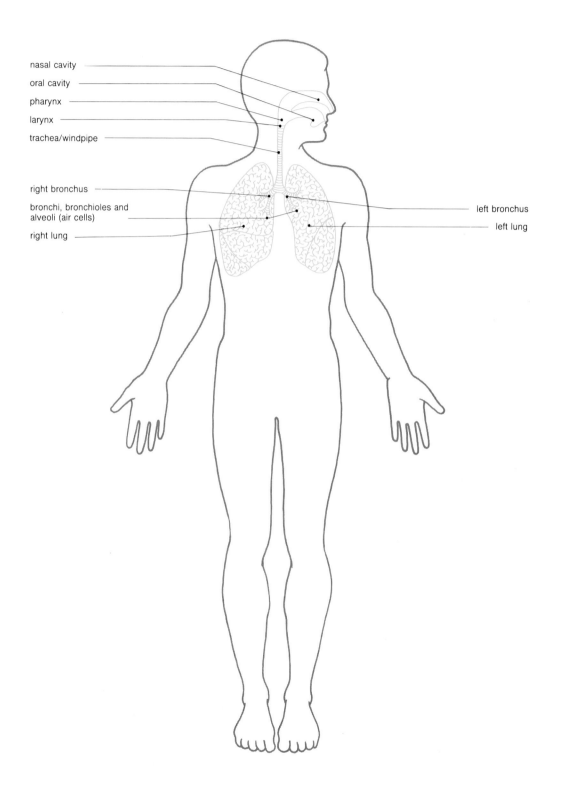

nasal cavity

oral cavity

pharynx

larynx

trachea/windpipe

right bronchus

bronchi, bronchioles and alveoli (air cells)

right lung

left bronchus

left lung

Glossary

Asana: Sitting place or posture to keep the body steady and relaxed, which is necessary for the practice of pranayama and meditation; yogic exercise for physical development and control.

Atman: The One Self; the Sole Reality or Brahman, which is ever pure, free, perfect and unchangeable; and which only exists in the body as a witness to all the changes in the body and mind.

Bandha: A muscular contraction which is sustained for a short period, sometimes to close the exits of the body, such as the windpipe or anus, thus preventing the escape of vital pranas, and assisting in sensory control and the raising of the Kundalini Shakti.

Bhakti yoga: That yoga path which seeks God-realisation (q.v.) through love and devotion to God.

Brahmacharya: Celibacy (sexual abstinence). Moderation in all spheres of life.

Brahma-jnana: Realisation of Brahman (God); the highest wisdom.

Brahman: God; the Absolute Reality, the Highest Being; the Ocean of Consciousness by Itself, the Ultimate Truth. Brahman is realised in the state of Nirvikalpa Samadhi (q.v.).

Chakra: "Wheel". Subtle seats of consciousness situated within the spinal column, which serve a number of psychosomatic functions. During the creation of the individual, the Kundalini Shakti, or central bodily power in man, descends through the sushumna nadi and leaves behind certain powers in the different chakras. In ordinary people the Kundalini Shakti stays in the lowest centre, muladhara chakra, situated between the anus and urethra. Here the Kundalini Shakti has taken its grossest form. During spiritual practice, the Kundalini Shakti tries to rise up through the sushumna nadi. When it rises fully to higher chakras, the energies of these chakras will be active, and the lower chakras will become inactive. In the three lowest chakras very low energies work, and the person will be attached to food, sleep and sex. In the fourth centre good energies work, but it is still not a permanent gain. Only when the Kundalini Shakti has risen fully above the fourth centre, is there a permanent spiritual gain, with no danger of a fall to lower sense pleasures. When the Kundalini Shakti rises fully to sahasrara in the crown of the head, Liberation is achieved. The six chakras are, starting with the lowest; muladhara chakra (the anus centre); swadhisthana chakra (at the level of the bladder); manipura chakra (at the level of the navel); anahata chakra (at the level of the heart); visuddha chakra (the throat centre), and ajna chakra (in the middle of the head). A seventh centre, the sahasrara or "thousand-petalled lotus" is situated in the crown of the head.

Chitta: "The mind stuff". In Vedanta psychology, chitta is one of the four functions of the mind (antah karana). In Swami Narayananda's psychology, chitta is the storehouse of all experiences, such as perceptions, inferences, passions, emotions and sentiments, from this and previous lives; chitta is Kundalini Shakti itself.

Dharana: Concentration of the mind on one point at will. The sixth stage of raja yoga (q.v.).

Dharma: The right or settled way of life; virtue and duty; the foundation for law and custom ensuring the well-being of society. Applicable to an individual as well as to a group or nation, and subject to time, place, age, position in society, and so on.

Dhyana: Meditation, deep contemplation. Prolonged concentration in dharana leads to this state. The seventh stage of raja yoga (q.v.).

God-realisation: To realise and become one with God. One may attain this state with form, Savikalpa Samadhi, or without form, Nirvikalpa Samadhi. Only in Nirvikalpa Samadhi does one return to the Absolute and become one with It.

Guru: A teacher or spiritual guide; especially one who gives initiation.

Hatha yoga: A branch of yoga for gaining control of the physical body and prana (q.v.), through physical and breathing exercises.

Ida: One of the subtle nerve channels or nadis (q.v.), through which the life force rises and descends. Situated outside and to the left of the spinal column, and running from muladhara to ajna chakra, where it joins the pingala nadi and sushumna, before descending to the left nostril.

Japa: Repeated repetition of God's name; especially of mantras, either verbally or mentally.

Jivatman: The individual soul.

Jnana yoga: The path leading to God or Self-Realisation through discrimination between the Real and the unreal.

Karma: Action. The theory of karma says that what one sows that one reaps (cf. Epistle to the Galatians 6:7), and that we are what our past thoughts, words and deeds have made us. Likewise we create our future by our present acts. The explanation is that all impressions of thoughts, words and deeds are kept in the chitta, and rise up to affect us in the future.

Karma phala: The fruit of past actions which we reap in the form of pleasure and pain.

Karma yoga: The yoga of selfless action; service to humanity without expectation of any reward.

Kriya: An act or process. A common term for purification methods.

Kumbhaka: Retention or suspension of breath.

Kundalini Shakti: The Primal Power in man, or the primordial cosmic energy; it is the energy source of all physical and mental functions. The rising up of this latent force through the chakras is the final aim of yoga. During the creation of the individual, Kundalini Shakti and the Self are separated, but only apparently, as they are one in reality. Kundalini Shakti descends to the lowest centre, the muladhara chakra, where it remains in most people. Partial risings of the Kundalini Shakti may, for instance, be caused by drugs or deep concentration. This is not a permanent attainment and may even be dangerous to one's spiritual development. When one engages in spiritual practices, or sadhana (q.v.), the Kundalini Shakti will try to rise upwards, but not until it goes fully above the heart centre is there no danger of a fall. When the Kundalini Shakti is reunited with its static centre in the sahasrara (q.v.), in the state of Nirvikalpa Samadhi, the person obtains Liberation and becomes one with the Ocean of Consciousness by Itself. Kundalini Shakti itself is chitta, i.e. the storehouse of all our past experiences from this and countless past lives. When we think, we get our past knowledge from chitta. The mind and the Kundalini Shakti interact. Mind gets its energy from the Kundalini Shakti to work in a dull or active way, so that the currents sent by the Kundalini Shakti to the body (like a dynamo, as it were) influence both the body and the mind. Kundalini Shakti is influenced by physical heat and cold, and by the qualities of the food one takes (e.g. heat-producing and cold-producing food).

Manas: According to classical Indian thought, manas is the mental faculty which compares, classifies and reasons, etc.

Mantra: Sacred syllables or a formula, repetition of which (either verbally or mentally), and reflection on which, purifies the mind and leads to real spiritual progress. A mantra is given by a guru.

Meditation: In general, deep thinking and serious contemplation and reflection. In the spiritual realm, meditation (dhyana) means deep thinking on the chosen form of God (ista).

Moksha or Mukti: Ultimate liberation, the goal and purpose of life according to yoga; deliverance from the "wheel of time", or the endless rounds of birth and death.

Mudras: Manual symbols shown with the hands; a certain class of yoga exercises, that aim at controlling the subtle energies of body and mind (prana q.v.).

Nadi: "Nerve". Nadis are both the physical nerves known from neuro-physiology, and subtler nerves that cannot be measured directly. The whole body is intertwined with nadis, through which nerve currents or Kundalini currents flow (cf. a similar idea in acupuncture). Some nadis are particularly important, e.g. ida and pingala (to the left and right of the spinal column respectively) and sushumna, which runs in the centre of the spinal column, and it is this nadi along which the chakras (q.v.) are situated.

Nirvana: Extinction of all desires, which results in liberation from the wheel of birth and death. Final emancipation. (See Moksha and Turiya.)

Nirvikalpa Samadhi: A superconscious state in which the individual consciousness merges in the Ocean of Consciousness by Itself, and where there is no mind or the triad, viz., subject, object and knowledge, or any idea whatever. In Nirvikalpa Samadhi, the Reality, Self or Brahman is apprehended, or realised.

Om: The Sacred Word designating Brahman, the All. It is the perfect word containing the full range of sounds of the human voice, and hence is known as the root mantra from whence all other mantras arise.

Pingala: The subtle nadi that is situated outside and to the right of the spinal column. (See Ida.)

Prana: Vital energy; nerve energy or life force. Prana is the main energy, and the source of all energies that work in the universe and in the body.

Pranayama: Breathing exercises that aim for mastery of the prana, and hence purification of the body, nadis and mind, to facilitate the rising of the Kundalini Shakti to higher centres.

Pratyahara: Withdrawal of the senses from their objects; the fifth step in raja yoga.

Puraka: Inspiration; inhalation of breath.

Raja yoga: That path which leads to Freedom through control of the mind, thoughts, desires and emotions. Raja yoga is traditionally divided into eight steps: 1. Yama (restraint), consisting of (a) ahimsa (non-violence, not to harm others in thought, word or deed); (b) satyam (truthfulness); (c) brahmacharya (celibacy); (d) asteyam (non-stealing) and (e) aparigraha (non-acceptance of luxurious gifts). 2. Niyama (observances), consisting of (a) saucha (purity); (b) santosha (contentment); (c) tapa (self-discipline, asceticism); (d) swadhyaya (study of holy scriptures) and (e) ishwara-pranidhana (devotion to and worship of God). In short, yama and niyama are the moral precepts that are found in all religions. 3. Asana (posture); in this context the right sitting posture for meditation. 4. Pranayama (breathing exercises). 5. Pratyahara (concentration), withdrawal of the senses from their object. 6. Dharana (concentration of the mind on one point at will). 7. Dhyana, "meditation" (a prolonging and deepening of dharana). 8. Samadhi (lit. "putting together", "synthesis"), the state in which the individual self is merged in the Universal Self or Brahman. In Savikalpa Samadhi, God is realised with form, and in Nirvikalpa Samadhi without form.

Rechaka: Exhalation of breath.

Sadhaka: Spiritual aspirant or truth seeker.

Sadhana: Steady and persevering practice of some method or exercise prescribed for spiritual ends.

Sahasrara: The uppermost centre (chakra) or "thousand-petalled lotus" situated in the crown of the head. When the Kundalini Shakti rises up fully to the sahasrara, Shiva and Shakti (Consciousness in its static and dynamic form) are united, and man becomes one with God.

Samadhi (lit. "putting together", "synthesis"): the state of super concentration in which the individual self is merged in the Universal Self or Brahman.

Samsara: The process of worldly life.

Samskaras: Residues in the mind left from past thinking and actions, which give rise, in each incarnation, to our mental and moral character.

Sanskrit: The classical language of North India; the oldest member of the Indo-European family, and the language in which the Vedas (the primary authority for all Hindus) are written.

Saraswati nadi: The fine nadi that, according to Swami Narayanananda, runs on the front side of the body connecting the brain with chitta in the muladhara chakra, and is used in all thought functions.

Savikalpa Samadhi: Realisation of God with form. In Savikalpa Samadhi, the soul still retains a certain awareness of itself as the "enjoyer", and the distinction between subject and object still exists for it.

Shakti: Force or energy. The Divine Power represented as the "female" principle, the "consort" of any deity.

Solar plexus: A complex of nerves situated in the abdomen.

Sushumna nadi: The finest of the yoga nadis situated within the spinal column and rising from the muladhara to the sahasrara and along which the chakras, or subtle seats of consciousness, are placed.

Tantras: Certain scriptures that have the form of a dialogue between Shiva and Shakti (his consort), and which constitute a set of rules for rituals, worship, discipline, meditation and the attainment of supernatural powers.

Trataka: Steady gazing; the process of fixing the gaze on a point for some time; a hatha yoga technique.

Turiya: The "fourth state" beyond waking, dreaming and deep sleep; the transcendental state of Pure Being, which no words can describe, since it transcends all individual experience. (See Moksha and Nirvana.)

Yantra: A symbolic diagram used for concentration.

Yoga (lit. "union"): Union with the Supreme Being, or of the lower and higher self. See under the different yoga paths: Bhakti yoga, Jnana yoga, Karma yoga and Raja yoga.

Yoga sutras: The classical Indian text on yoga; attributed to Patanjali, c. second century B.C.

Yogi: One who practises yoga.

Bibliography

Anatomy and physiology
J.R. McClintic: *Human Anatomy,* C.V. Mosby Co., Missouri, 1983
H.O. Kendall, F.P. Kendall and G.E. Wadsworth: *Muscles, Testing and Function,* Williams and Wilkins, Baltimore/London, 1983

Diet and nutritional physiology
Rudolf Ballentine: *Diet and Nutritional Therapy,* Himalayan Institute, Pennsylvania, 1978
Linda Clark: *Know Your Nutrition,* Keats Pubs., Texas, 1984.
Dr. C.C. Shears: *Nutrition Science and Health Education,* The Nutrition Science Research Institute of England, Gloucester, 1978

Body consciousness and therapy
R. Anderson: *Stretching,* Shelter Pubs., California, 1980
Daniels and Worthingham: *Muscle Testing,* W.B. Saunders, Philadelphia, 1980
R.A. McKenzie: *The Lumbar Spine,* Spinal Pubs., New Zealand, 1981
John B. West: *Respiratory Physiology: the Essentials,* Williams and Wilkins, Baltimore/London, 1979

Hatha yoga, pranayama and relaxation
Theos Bernard: *Hatha yoga,* Rider, London 1982
B.K.S. Iyengar: *Light on Pranayama,* George Allen and Unwin, London, 1981
B.K.S. Iyengar: *Light on Yoga,* George Allen and Unwin, London, 1968. Reprinted 1985.

Swami Kuvalyananda: *Asanas, Popular Prakashan,* Bombay, 1981
Swami Kuvalyananda: *Pranayama, Popular Prakashan,* Bombay, 1981
Swami Narayanananda: *The Secrets of Prana, Pranayama and Yoga Asanas,* N.U. Yoga Ashrama, Denmark, 1979
Pancham Sinh: *The Hatha Yoga Pradipika,* Oriental Books Reprint Corp., New Delhi, 1980
Rai Bahadur Srisa Chandra Vasa: *The Gheranda Samhita,* Sri Satguru Pubs., New Delhi, 1981

Yoga psychology, philosophy and meditation
Swami Hariharananda Aranya: *Yoga Philosophy of Patanjali,* State University of New York Press, Albany, 1983
Swami Balakrishnananda: *Yogic Depth Psychology,* N.U. Yoga Ashrama, Denmark, 1980
Swami Narayanananda: *The Secrets of Mind-Control,* N.U. Yoga Ashrama, Denmark, 1979
Swami Narayanananda: *The Primal Power in Man or The Kundalini Shakti:* N.U. Yoga Ashrama, Denmark, 1979
Swami Narayanananda: *The Mysteries of Man, Mind and Mind-Functions,* N.U. Yoga Ashrama, Denmark, 1979
Swami Swarupananda: *Srimad Bhagavad Gita,* Advaita Ashrama, India, 1981